I0569211

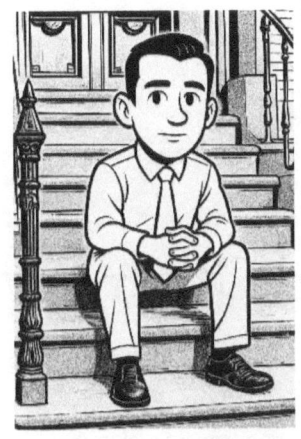

About the Author

Asher Lockwood is a healer and an addict. He's been addicted to drugs, sex, work, fame, money and power. From Yale to jail, Asher, a former Psychiatric Nurse Practitioner and CEO, spent 6 years in a horrifically abusive relationship with a truly sociopathic stripper all while suffering active Bipolar Type I with psychosis. He is currently an active father to two boys, engaged to a beautiful stable, drug-free woman, spends time with his family, has his friends back, and is substance-free, loving every day that he's here and present. A pattern of bad decisions has landed him on track for federal prison, with sentencing set for November 15, 2025. He would rather serve his whole prison sentence than spend another day with his dreaded ex-wife Aileen.

This is his first book, written without the benefit of treatment for his severe ADHD. While on probation, he spent countless hours at the local library, sifting through a clouded mind to piece together the brutal saga of his suffering and survival, still wondering how he's made it this far. He hopes that by turning his pain into purpose, his story might light the way for others facing similar struggles. With life experience second to none, he now shares his story.

"Here in the darkness, I know myself, can't break free until I let it go, let me go" - Amy Lee

Adderall and Other False Prophets:

How Mental Illness and Addiction Derailed a Psychiatric CEO's Million-Dollar Mind

By

Asher Lockwood

Copyright

Disclaimer

This memoir is a personal recollection of events and conversations and is presented to the best of the author's memory. Certain names, identifying details, and locations have been changed or withheld to protect the privacy of individuals. Some persons, places, and incidents portrayed herein may be composite or fictionalized; any resemblance to actual persons, living or dead, or actual events is intentional only where explicitly noted. This work is provided for informational and entertainment purposes only and does not constitute professional advice; the author and publisher assume no liability for any errors, omissions, or any outcomes arising from the use of the information contained herein.

Copyright © 2025 by Asher Lockwood. All rights reserved. No part of this book may be used or reproduced by any means, graphic, electronic, or mechanical, including photocopying, recording, taping, or by any information storage retrieval system, without the written permission of the publisher except in the case of brief quotations embodied in reviews.

Name: Lockwood, Asher, 1982-author.
Title: Adderall and Other False Prophets: How Mental Illness and Addiction Derailed a Psychiatric CEO's Million-Dollar Mind / Asher Lockwood.
Identifiers: LCCN 2025916318 | ISBN 979-8-9931032-4-2 (Trade Paperback)
Classification: DDC 362.29/9092[B]-dc23
This book may be purchased in bulk for promotional, educational, or business use. Please contact your local bookseller or Dark Prism Press by email.
Published by Dark Prism Press 2025
2248 Broadway New York, NY 10024

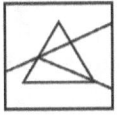

Acknowledgements

To my parents for providing both Lorenzo and I with a great childhood

To my two sons, Giovanni & Lorenzo, you mean the world to me

To J.B. and family, thank you for helping my son when it mattered the most

To P.D. and the double Windsor knot, you will always be in my heart, thank you

To Judge D., in anticipation of your mercy

To my brother, you will always be an important part of my life

To the Stiz crew, you know who you are, nothing but love

To James B., brother in arms

To Abbie, for having been a fantastic spouse and exceptional mother to Giovanni

To Dr. Karens, for always being there when needed

To Dr. N., for not giving up on me and encouraging me to write this book

To Elle, for always staying with me through the storm

To my guardian angels, Jeanne M. & Dottie W., you are very missed

To those I lost along the way, especially Adam N, to drugs and alcohol

To Elle, again, I wouldn't be here if it wasn't for you

Introduction

My world went up in an inferno, and I stood amid the ashes, head genuflecting in regret. How had I, a board-certified psychiatric nurse practitioner and CEO, lost everything, and the one person who meant more than life itself? This is the story of rediscovering the man beneath the facade and titles.

Over six brutal years, I battled a perfect storm of addiction, spiraling mental illness, and a toxic marriage to a sociopathic partner, while trying to protect two little boys caught in the crossfire. Family court hearings, inpatient stays, and a symphony of rehab programs along the way offered only temporary relief. Every mistake cut deeper than the last, teaching me painful lessons I never wanted to comprehend but had to face and understand.

Not even my medical training at Yale or years in psychiatric practice could have prepared me for this fall from grace, or the excruciatingly bone-deep torment I would endure clawing my way out of that hole. Stripped of my freedom, my career, and my sense of self, I discovered that true mastery begins within the very place we are so afraid to look: deep inside ourselves.

Join me on this raw, unflinching journey into self-discovery, resilience and redemption. You'll see how knowing yourself – down to your very core – becomes the ultimate lifeline. Through grit, self-compassion, and the unwavering support of others, we can transform our darkest moments into the greatest triumphs.

This is my story. May it inspire you to reclaim your own.

DEA Raid

On a Tuesday morning in January 2024, my life changed again, following the pattern of chaos I'd found myself trapped in for the past seven years. The last few days had been filled with crushing news from family court, arguments with my girlfriend, and a physical altercation with my housemate, so I was eager to return to the routine of the work week. In addition to running a successful private psychiatry practice, I was also in the process of launching a concierge mobile IV infusion business.

I unlocked the door to my rented office and gathered the mail that the building owner had slipped under the door. I shuffled through the envelopes, the usual mix of junk, referrals from primary care physicians, and record requests. I stepped into the adjoined waiting room/reception area and dropped the request for medical records on my office manager's desk so she could scan the files and fax them over. The first patient wouldn't be arriving for another hour, giving us time to prepare for what seemed so far like a normal clinical day.

Suddenly, a man stepped into the waiting room and asked if he could speak with me for a minute. He wasn't a patient, but I recognized him: Mr. Bryant, the DEA agent who, a little over a year earlier, had stopped by the house of Aileen's (my soon-to-be-ex-wife) father, where I had been living at the time. The original visit seemed to be harmless, supposedly just confirming my address since I had moved around quite a bit in the years prior. Aileen had acted strangely in front of the agent and nervously refused to give him her cell phone number, which I thought was odd. I took Mr. Bryant's business card, and he left the house.

My second encounter with him was in October 2023. I separated from Aileen in September, and I was set to attend the wedding of my friend Craig. Aileen knew about the wedding and, in an attempt to punish me for not bringing her (even though we were separated), she bombarded me with text messages claiming Mr. Bryant had stopped by her father's house again looking for me. She texted me a photo of his business card as "proof". I went through my wallet and realized the business card he had given me the year before at the original visit was missing. Always planning her next manipulations and leverage points, I realized Aileen must have stolen it from my wallet at some point to use against me in the future. I put her out of my mind and enjoyed the wedding.

Although I assumed she was lying (and she was), I made the decision to reach out to Mr. Bryant preemptively. I let him know via email my current office location, contact information, and asked him if he had been trying to contact me as I was currently going through a messy separation and Aileen said he stopped by. I wanted to get on paper with them that she was angry and vindictive in case she tried to contact them again. Mr. Bryant called me and confirmed that she was lying: "Brother, I wasn't even in the state of New York that day."

But this visit, in January, felt different than all prior contacts with him. He pulled me into my office and began asking me questions about my e-prescribing software, how controlled substances were sent to pharmacies, and for the records of two specific patients. I didn't have the records; the patients were remnants of a recent former life I was trying to get away from. Upon my failure to produce the records, Mr. Bryant excused himself to supposedly retrieve a form for me to fill out regarding the missing information. When he returned, he was joined by about a dozen DEA agents with guns and vests, who immediately handcuffed me and my office manager and began tearing the office apart in a frenzy.

Their search yielded nothing, and I was forced to stand in the main hallway of the office building in handcuffs for what felt like forever, in full view of the other building tenants. The agents sorted all paperwork from my office, as well as our computers and phones, into sealed evidence bags. I was then escorted to the agents' vehicle.

What happened after this is a blur. I was put into the custody of US Marshals, then brought to a federal courthouse for a hearing. The Judge didn't think I was in the right mindset, whatever the "right mindset" would be in this situation, and I was sent to jail for the next three days. I can't remember most of the hearing, besides the prosecutor's words that I was facing "25 to life" echoing in my head.

The US Marshals then took me to the jail, and I was stripped down for intake. I handed over my street clothes, and I became scared at the prospect that I would never see them again. Next, I was scanned for metal and inspected for contraband before being sent to a cell. I was put in a cell alone, as my mental illness preceded me. The next three days were harrowing, as I detoxed from Klonopin as well as withdrew from 10 psychotropic medications.

It wasn't always like this. Once upon a time, I was literally on top of the world, with a massive empire that spanned coast to coast. But my current predicament was just the culmination of years of addiction, mental illness, domestic abuse, bad decisions, and being in the wrong place at the wrong time. This is my fall from grace. This is my story.

Steady Breath, Steady Gaze

The expectations for my life were set before I took my first breath. As the first-born male in a Sicilian family, it was ingrained in me from a young age that I needed to be a worthy heir to the family name. My father, the "enforcer" of the family, was an extremely brilliant and successful dentist, highly esteemed and commanding a healthy income. My mother, once a pediatric nurse, left her job to fulfill her beloved maternal role to myself and my younger brother. While it wasn't assumed that I would follow exactly in my father's footsteps as a dentist, I was expected to be successful. I remember my father's words: "I don't care if you're a rocket scientist or a garbageman but be the best one you can be" (with the unspoken implication that he hoped I tended closer to the former). Growing up, the emphasis in my household was always on intellectual and financial attainment. The bar was high and they never let me forget it. But things like being called "boy idiot" while growing up didn't help my confidence. This all ended up weighing heavily on me, an unfortunate complement to the mental illness that would end up grabbing hold of my life.

My first tangle with panic attacks came at age ten. Of course, being a kid, I didn't recognize it at the time as a "panic attack," but I'll never forget it. My family and I were on vacation at Disney World. We had just returned to our hotel room after a long day at the parks and my parents wanted to go on a walk alone, so they left me in charge of watching my little brother. The scene is burned into my mind: the door swinging shut behind my parents as they left, the blinding lights of the suite, the two twin beds, the smell of individually wrapped hotel room soap, the baseball game on the TV. Suddenly, terror hit me like a wave. I ran to the balcony, hoping to see my parents below. My view was entirely blocked by palm trees. My throat tightened. My heart was pounding, I couldn't catch my breath. What was this high-pitched ringing in my ears? *What if they were never coming back?* I thought. *Or worse, what if they're dead??*

I darted from the balcony to the hotel room door and back again. Had it been minutes, or hours? My brother was lying on the bed, simply watching my frantic behavior. With each passing second, I became increasingly sure that we'd be on our own forever and never see our parents again. My eyes landed on the phone between the two beds. I picked up the receiver with trembling hands and dialed the front desk.

Suddenly, a voice rang out on the other end. The woman listened to my panic-stricken story of my parents leaving for a walk and disappearing forever, and miraculously, she understood. She kept my mind busy, telling me the "secret" of how the parks don't *really* close at night, the staff work underground in secret tunnels to service everything and prepare for guests the next day. I was enraptured by this insider knowledge as her kind voice kept me distracted long enough for time to return to normal speed. Before I knew it, my parents had returned from their walk. Immediately, my breathing returned to normal and my heart stopped racing. As if a switch was flipped, my panic completely dissipated.

This hidden fear, my separation anxiety-fueled panic, continued as I hit puberty. Whenever my parents went out for a date night, I was riddled with fear. Fortunately, as I entered my teen years, I was able to gradually grow out of panic attacks for a little bit by gravitating toward my group of friends. This allowed me a level of stability and a brief respite from the searing fear that threatened to engulf my mind as I entered high school.

I attended Catholic school through eighth grade. I entered public high school in the suburban Connecticut town of Saddlebrooke where I grew up. I enjoyed my time in high school, getting a B+ average, staying active with sports, attaining a level of popularity, and earning myself the nickname 'The Lock'. My first steady long-term girlfriend was Sarah, whom I dated for almost four years. Although she was in the grade below me, we spent plenty of time together (probably too much, verging on enmeshment, if I'm being perfectly honest).

My senior year of high school was by far my favorite. I had a great group of friends, Sarah, and somewhat of an urban legend hero status (not before getting an *extremely* stern talking-to from my father, as the notoriety came from an experience where Sarah and I skipped school to hook up and were unexpectedly interrupted by her mother's voice just outside the bathroom door, leading to me jumping out the second story window and running half-naked through a funeral). Somehow, I managed to stay out of trouble long enough to graduate and gain acceptance to

Adderall and Other False Prophets

Fairfield University, my family's alma mater for the past two generations. An hour away, it was far enough for a new start, but not so far as to be anxiety-provoking or lead me too far from my hometown friends.

At the prospective University freshman overnight event, I met the kid who would become my first roommate, Nikolaos. It was that night that I smoked weed for the first time. I quickly became disoriented and, even though I had been having fun up until that point, asked Nikolaos to escort me back to my room. The experience had rendered me unable to socialize with anyone or participate in the evening activities. Do people *enjoy* feeling like this? It made no sense to me at the time. It would be my first brush with drugs, but definitely not the last.

Nikolaos and I roomed together freshman year in Dolan Hall. Our next-door neighbor was Michael, who I technically met on the campus network (he had the most porn available and uploaded). Michael and I quickly became best friends, and I knew we would be boys for life. We hit it off from the get-go, a crazy Italian and an Irishman. We rolled together just about everywhere.

A nunnery converted into a snug dorm, Dolan was rumored to be haunted because a pregnant nun and the priest who impregnated her had supposedly hanged themselves there years before. There were certainly creepy noises in the stairwells, especially near the old church. However, I had little time for investigating paranormal occurrences as I was too busy getting high on pot (I ended up giving it another chance, with much better results) and trying to attend my pre-med biology lectures.

It was at these lectures that Abbie first caught my eye. The gem of the freshman class, she was beautiful, charismatic, incredibly smart, and out of my league. From the first moment I saw her, I made it my mission to have her. But it soon became apparent that I was basically nobody compared to all the senior boys showering her with attention. Despite this small setback, freshman year ended on a high note and I was back in my hometown of Saddlebrooke for the summer of a lifetime.

Polarity Blossoms

The summer of 2001 was like no other and I was on full tilt, living every second to the fullest. After a freshman year spent experimenting with freedom and gateway drugs, I was ready for a summer of debauchery: drinking, smoking, cars, girls, the boys, etc. *The Fast and the Furious* had just come out, leading my friends and I to deck out our whips and hit the parties (I had a brand-new Nissan Pathfinder, which I kept immaculate...except for when I would take it off-roading and ended up covered in mud. That's what car washes are for, right?). I was the leader of the pack, the king of Saddlebrooke, at least in my own manic mind. Nothing could stop me or slow me down. It wasn't until many years later that I fully understood what happened to me that summer.

I was working three jobs: mailman in the morning, waiter in the afternoon, and partier in the evening. My days started at 5:00 a.m. sorting mail and ended at 2:00 or 3:00 a.m. in friends' basements, stoned, drunk, laughing, watching movies, and playing pool, with girls in tow. My soon-to-be-ex Sarah had hooked us up with her cousin, a weed dealer from the next town over who only had the good shit. We kicked off every night at his house at around 7:00 p.m. and ended every night absolutely rocked on kush, driving home at about 20 mph. We always made it home safe; we were invincible.

My energy radiated around me and everyone gravitated towards me. I was getting only two or three hours of sleep a night but felt completely normal. Hot girls who wouldn't give me the time of day in high school were suddenly texting me nonstop and showering me with attention like it was going out of style. My reputation exploded. Nothing could slow me down (believe me, my parents tried like their lives depended on it). Suddenly, there wasn't enough of me to go around. Even the jocks recognized my rising authority in the social scene of our town.

Just when it seemed like I had already fully capitalized on my newfound contagious positive energy, I decided to throw a party. I wanted it to be the Rager to end all Ragers. The jewel in the crown of my golden social status, this night was going to be crazy. I wanted it to be the kind of party people talked about for years, and I certainly succeeded. My friends and I had everything planned weeks in

13

advance. Everything came together perfectly when my parents announced they were leaving for Maine for a week and taking my brother with them. I was staying home to "work and take care of the house".

My family backed out of the driveway and my crew got to work. Ten 30 racks, drugs, munchies, music, girls. Dozens of people began to show up. Earlier, Sarah and I had gotten into a fight (the kind that ends relationships), so I was surprised to see that even she dared to make an appearance. Not only that, but word had gotten around about the party and most of her graduating class came too. Soon, my entire cul-de-sac was flooded with cars and people started parking on neighboring streets. My two best friends from high school lived on either side of me and helped escort people to and from their cars to avoid getting the cops called. Although I was grateful for the help, I wasn't even worried about the situation in the first place. I wasn't afraid of the cops! No one could slow down my momentum.

The party roared on as I wandered the halls to check everything out, my energy buzzing around me. Kids were ripping nitrous in my living room. Raucous drinking games were being played in the kitchen and rec room. *Are those two girls making out on my dad's recliner?* Music blasted everywhere. *Why is Michael smoking a cigarette in the house??!* Dudes were high fiving me and slapping me on the back, girls pressed against me in the hallways as they shot me suggestive glances. All the most popular guys and hottest girls from both graduating classes were in my house, partying and having a great time. Even girls I had met on vacation had shown up, drawn to the party due to my newfound reputation. I had arrived and come into my own. When it was time to rest, I kicked out the partygoers having a threesome in my bed and took Sarah with me as my queen (mostly because she wouldn't leave me alone the whole evening, scaring off the other potentials).

*   *   *

The next day was something out of a movie. Inevitably, my house was destroyed, so my friends and I quickly formed a cleanup crew. It took us about six days and $3000.00 in supplies and repairs to get everything passable again. Good thing I had all this energy! On the day my family was due to come home, I made sure

I was out of the house and doing something they would approve of (fishing with one of my best friends).

"Come home." The text message from my father flashed on my cell phone screen. He never said much, but when he did, it was serious. I drove home in silence, wondering what awaited me. When I arrived, he pulled me into a room alone and told me that he knew I had "at least fifteen people over" while they were gone. Let me repeat that: my parents had determined that the massive party was "fifteen people." I had never been so happy to hear anything in my life. I immediately hung my head in shame and said quietly, "You're right, Dad" before apologizing profusely. I had gotten away with having about 200 additional people over that he never found out about, thanks to my friends' and my hard work for a week straight on almost no sleep. Cell phones didn't have cameras yet (let's hear it for the Nokia 5110!) and social media wasn't a thing, so any photographic proof to the contrary was languishing away in the depths of someone's digital camera. Years later, I would end up telling him the truth about that night. He still couldn't believe it.

*   *   *

With only one month left in the summer of 2001, my friends and I wanted to make the most of it. To us, that meant smoking weed for thirty days straight before the big return to college to begin our sophomore year. By the end of August, we could barely remember anything, let alone string together coherent sentences. It was the perfect chill way to end the perfect summer. As I arrived back on campus, I excitedly thought about how I would be rooming with my partner in crime, Michael.

Due to a stroke of luck, Michael and I had both scored high on the dorm lottery and therefore had the first choice of rooms. I made sure we were in the same hall as my major crush, Abbie. After running into our RA, who we knew and realized would basically let us get away with murder, we immediately began to set up shop. Our first order of business, the one I had been waiting for, was to go one floor up and down the hall to the girls' wing where Abbie would be living. Seeing her again after the long summer filled me with warm feelings.

Adderall and Other False Prophets

Abbie and I grew very close that semester. One evening, on the tennis courts against the backdrop of the setting sun, Abbie and I made a joint decision to change our majors from pre-med to nursing. My circle quickly tightened to Michael and Abbie, and amidst the straining demands of my new major, I quickly began to feel isolated compared to the buzzing summer I had just experienced. I suddenly found myself a king without a throne.

Michael was predisposed to alcoholism and depression, things I previously knew nothing about. But I soon found myself in the merciless grip of depression and anxiety as my mental health began to decompensate. It started with a tightening in my chest, the rush of invisible danger, a mind racing toward catastrophe with no clear threat in sight. My fear center was completely lit up, signaling me to try and outrun something I couldn't see. Panic. I wound up experiencing my first panic attack since that one all those years ago on vacation. But this time, it was different, more visceral. My heart was pounding, the collar of my shirt was drenched in sweat, what was happening? I felt myself falling into this dark abyss where all fears come true. What should I do?! My eyes scanned every inch of the room. Linkin Park's "In the End" music video was playing on the TV and it pulled me in while my brain cooked in overdrive.

Thank God Michael was there to identify what was happening and talk me down. Once I knew that I wasn't dying, I calmed down slightly. I learned that day to recognize and acknowledge the presence of panic in order to get through it. You can't fight it; the harder you fight it, the stronger it becomes. It literally becomes fear of fear. Panic attacks actually speed the brain up just like seizures and it takes time to wind down. Once it's over, you feel like you have just finished running a marathon. I had never felt so bad in my life and never wanted to experience that again. Unfortunately, that attack was just the foot in the door for darker experiences.

As things got worse for me, I tried to establish myself through Abbie but kept falling through the cracks. Where was the boundless energy I had over the summer? I could no longer survive on a couple hours of sleep, and the once-reliable waves of energy I counted on to propel me through long days of partying and work were long gone. In fact, I was now sleeping every day for at least twelve hours, often until the afternoon. I was skipping class at an alarming frequency. The sudden unfathomable lows I was experiencing stood in contrast so stark to the sunny highs of the summer that it gave me whiplash. Abbie tried her best to help me; aside from the huge crush I had on her, she was also an incredible friend. She would show up every day and try to drag my ass to class. If it wasn't for her, I probably would have failed out of school that year.

*   *   *

The ability to make a conscious decision depends on one's realization of their situation. There's the self you always knew, and then there's the self you come to know with mental illness. When I became an adult, I always thought I had a good idea of who I was as a person. But breaking bipolar at age nineteen kind of threw things off course for me. To continue in college, survive, and prosper, I needed to find a way to accept and live with this newfound disease. At first, I tried fighting with it, trying to identify and deal with the symptoms individually. I went into an avoidant state; anything not to feel the pain again of panic, sleep problems, depression, and drug abuse. Every day, I woke up wondering if I would go to class, be able to interact with others, if I could get the grades my parents were expecting me to get. Then, the anxiety took me over. Instead of focusing on academics or my social life, I became preoccupied with being sick. I became an identified patient. I was sick and required rescue.

In some ways, Abbie ended up pulling me out of my bipolar break that year. My relationship with her was blossoming. We began the year as inseparable friends but ended the first semester as a fused couple. I'll never forget the magical visit I had with her over the winter break of that year. We took a train ride to visit New York City, see the big tree, explore, and admire the sparkling lights that adorned every city building. We walked around and eventually ended up in Bryant Park. Sitting on a wall and enjoying each other's company, I pulled a small gift out of my pocket and handed it to her. She unwrapped the beautiful diamond necklace, adorned with a small cross, and loved it. Her eyes lit up. That's when I told her "I love you" for the first time. She didn't immediately return the sentiment, but she did later that night. We caught the night train back to her Upstate New York family home and spent the night together. My world was absolutely glowing; I felt so safe in that moment.

With Abbie by my side, the rest of the year seemed to go relatively smoothly, with my mental illness symptoms only increasing towards the end of the school year. No one knew what my diagnosis was yet and wouldn't for some time. I was put on Zoloft, which worked for about six months. When the meds stopped working and weed wasn't helping, my relationship with Abbie filled the void. She had shown me mercy when I needed it the most, so I held onto her with a death grip. She was my safety.

I didn't realize it at the time, but I was cross-addicted: to drugs and to Abbie. She was the better choice; when we were together, it felt like I didn't need drugs. I tried to serve her as best I could because she had saved me from the true abyss. When I was alone, my life felt dark and troubled. When I was with Abbie, my life felt warm and alive, and my days were filled with social excursions and parties with people who previously wouldn't have looked at me twice. We traveled extensively with both her family and mine, to Maine, Italy, and Florida. Everyone got along so well, it was like it was meant to be.

At this point, the new me was a combination of Abbie and bipolar symptoms. This became a comfortable and acceptable narrative for me to adopt as a nineteen-year-old; it helped me navigate my mental illness the best I could. I left myself behind, stopped maturing and differentiating, and lived this superficial narrative. I didn't realize at the time that this 'Teenage Asher' would continue to live on within me from this point forward. Between my enmeshment with Abbie and my new identity as a mental health patient, I ceased to differentiate as an individual and now had a new identity within the confines of our relationship.

*   *   *

Life continued on campus. At night, Michael and I would carry out insane schemes, like selling a pound of pot (he ended up smoking all of his), stealing a common area plasma TV (even though we wore stockings over our faces, we still got so paranoid that we threw the TV in the river and never spoke of it again), and breaking into a vending machine at 3:30 a.m. (we were unsuccessful but did manage to burn a hole in the floor using hydrochloric acid). Mostly we just did drugs, which exacerbated the decline of our fragile mental states. Unbeknownst to me, he was even smoking black tar and opium frequently. He rarely got off the futon in our dorm room. I even once accidentally picked up the bong he was using to smoke, not knowing that it had opium in it, and didn't realize my mistake until I noticed the strange taste. I won't say I didn't enjoy it; Michael and I sat facing each other and had an incredible four-hour-long philosophical discussion on life. But it wasn't something I wanted to do again. It turns out he had been taking a cab into the east side of Bridgeport (straight-up gang territory) to get that shit.

I just want to point something out here: if an addict wants to do drugs, they will always find a way. Michael, without money, transportation, or a hook-up for the dope, decided to take a cab to a dangerous area, ask around for black tar or opium, and paid for it using cash he made from pawning his stuff. He successfully hid these missions from me, and we shared a ten-by-eight-foot room, for God's sake! The cab ride alone, one way, would have been at least $30.00 at that time. Addicts, including myself, will do anything. Do not forget that.

Michael dropped out of college junior year because he wasn't doing well and ended up getting an apartment in Bridgeport. It was in an extremely dangerous part of town, infamous for widespread gang and cartel activity. Nearby, there were government housing buildings with some very non-government "armed guards" wielding AK-47s to keep people out. We heard that you could buy anything there: dope, guns, stolen cars, even trafficked humans. To afford the place, he took in two drug dealers as roommates. They were nice guys, but they were peddling some serious shit.

Naturally, we decided one night to roll up to a strip club in the heart of the east side. Blasting 50 Cent's "I'm Supposed To Die Tonight" from my brand-new Acura MDX, we arrived at the club and parked behind an Escalade on thirty-inch rims. When we arrived at the door, the bouncer actually had a look of concern on his face. He must have thought we were insane. Somehow, he let us in and we sat down at the bar and ordered Heinekens. We looked over to the pool table to see a guy with a cane, top hat, glasses, and an actual white fur coat with his crew staring back at us.

A stripper sat down next to us and asked if we were lost. I lit up and replied, "No, baby doll, what can I do for you?" She ordered a Baileys on the rocks, costing me ten dollars (it was a rip-off, but I paid anyway to satisfy the atmosphere of the club). Surprisingly, Michael and I had a great time that night, and no one fucked with us. They probably figured that the crazy Italian and Irishman either knew someone or were truly insane. Michael even ended up banging one of the girls in a booth for $75.00.

That wasn't the only crazy situation we found ourselves in. Two weeks before my 21st birthday, I got caught with a fake ID at a liquor store right near campus. Now, what you need to know is that the Clam Jam was going on at the beach front. This celebration is a reason for the entire student body to spill out onto the beach and party like there's no tomorrow. *Everyone* was there. So, after being arrested I was cuffed and searched by police on the spot, right in full view of the entire student body. I was dying of embarrassment as the cop held me up against a squad car in front of a wall of thousands of my peers. I swear it felt like the music and crowd noise went silent as everyone stared at me.

After I was released, I immediately got a $2500.00 lawyer. I didn't have the full amount, so Michael lent me $1500.00 (which I never actually paid back, but I always took care of him whenever we went out on the town, so it probably evened out). I got the charge dropped but had to do community service at the local YMCA. I never told my parents what had happened. They questioned my "volunteering," and I told them I was just being nice and giving back to the community (yeah, right...). They somehow fell for it and I was off the hook.

I spent a ton of time with Michael in the coming months. Being in Tremont, he had access to a ton of drugs and we spent every weekend and most weekdays completely lit. He eventually gave up the tar (but kept everything else). Despite the drugs and the mental issues that continued to overshadow my life, I was somehow able to keep up my grades. Abbie and I excelled in nursing and we graduated from Fairfield in 2004 with honors, ready to begin a career that would hopefully carry us the rest of our lives.

*   *   *

After graduation, Abbie and I were accepted into Yale New Haven Hospital to work as bedside nurses, myself in the surgical ICU and Abbie in the medical ICU. This was a huge honor for both of us, and we got an apartment together about ten minutes away in East Haven. The surgical ICU was a big deal, housing very high-profile surgeries and using new technologies that were on the cutting edge of medicine, like the Da Vinci surgical robot. It was incredible that I, a new first-year grad, was hired for the SICU. I was to work for a six-month orientation period as sort of an intern before becoming autonomous. Yale was extremely serious, and the expectations placed upon RNs seemed to be even higher than those for medical residents.

I met some of the smartest, most renowned people I would ever know at Yale. I bonded the most with Dr. Jeffrey Craw, an attending. He was a trauma surgeon out of Chicago who was now rising to the top of the ranks at Yale. He understood that the nurses really ran the SICU (we ran codes and could do everything except intubation) and basically dictated the residents to fill the orders we issued. Jeff was also a tenth-degree black belt and could wield a sword like no other. We got along very well, mostly because I was an extremely hard worker and always eager to gain more knowledge. He even catered to me every time I came into work vomiting because I was "dehydrated" (having a panic attack), taking me off assignment and directing a fellow to hang an IV bag of Lactated Ringer's solution for me. This was a massive help; the psychosomatic component of mental illness is very real and I actually did suffer terrible diarrhea and vomiting at times (of course, it was totally in my head and I would feel fine and even hungry the second I got off my shift, but it certainly made work a nightmare).

One day, Jeff told me the story of how he found himself. Prior to med school, he drove cross-country on a motorcycle. In Illinois, he met a gentleman at a bar who explained to him how *he*, too, found himself. Jeff had absorbed every word. I think he was telling me this to get me to realize that I still needed to attain self-actualization. He was right, but I didn't see it at the time. What was there to find? I was a nurse in the Yale New Haven SICU; I was a big shot. I already had it all figured out! Or at least that's what I told myself to avoid having to deal with the reality: I was scared, mentally ill, fully enmeshed with my girlfriend, and I still hadn't mentally progressed past age nineteen. As long as I kept busy, I thought that I could outrun myself.

Both Abbie and I worked the night shift, on opposite nights. When she worked 7:00 p.m.-7:00 a.m., I would either go down to Bridgeport to visit Michael or he would come to visit me. We would usually either hit the clubs or the huge casino about half an hour away. We'd spend dumb amounts of money, his from selling drugs and mine from my nursing job. Sometimes our other friends would tag along, and we'd pick up some girls. Michael, being a literal genius (he could have joined MENSA if he wanted to, but he was smart enough to know better), could accurately count cards. After making off with some hefty sums of cash, he was eventually caught and brought into a backroom by two unmarked guards. We were summarily banned from the casino under threat of arrest. That was fine with us; we had all our limbs and the cash we had scored over the past few weeks, and we were out!

Michael and I would also occasionally take advantage of our relatively high incomes and geographic proximity to NYC. We would hop on the train to the city to meet up with friends, go to cooler clubs, and do tons of cocaine. The drug had grown in popularity within our friend group now that we had grown-up money, so there was always an eight ball or two amongst our crew when we went out. Yes, it was stomped, but whose shit isn't? I was always willing to pay more if it was right off the block. Sometimes I wish I could go back to the 80's, just to experience what coke was like back then.

One weekend, Abbie had gone home to visit family, and us boys went to the city. The four of us got a hotel room in Manhattan and a ridiculous amount of coke. We were pregaming in the hotel room when Dr. Cohen collapsed after doing too much. He had literally hoovered over the entire pile like a fiend! He and I were the only ones in the room with medical training, and he certainly wasn't in any position to provide care for himself. I sprang into action, hanging an IV for him to get him back on his feet and ready to hit the clubs.

Lockwood

That night we decided to go to 1 Oak, one of the nicer clubs in Manhattan. By the time we got through the line and to the door, we had to cough up $1500.00 just for a table. We paid without a second thought and were escorted to our table. The girls were hot and dressed to the nines. All I'll say here is that we spent stupid money (the $1500.00 covered the first round of drinks only) and got back to the hotel around 5:00 a.m.. We got back to the room and I hung more IVs for everyone to minimize the damage before passing out. A few hours later, I woke to see one of the guys sitting on the end of the bed with a cheap prostitute in front of him. Dumbass was sharing our candy supply with her! I quickly put an end to that. Despite all that happened that weekend, it was an awesome time and a great memory I'll always share with Michael and the guys.

Michael and I had tons more adventures in the next couple of years, usually including strip clubs, girls, drugs, gambling, tons of clove cigarettes, and just general partying. He'll always be my best friend and I'll never forget all the great times we shared. Unfortunately, my life at this point wasn't all partying and living it up.

Death's Delicate Dance

March 23, 2005, was a night that I'll never forget. I was living at home and had just come off of a stint of four straight night shifts in a row. My father came into my room and woke me up. My mother had severe abdominal pain and was in the emergency room in the local podunk hospital. He couldn't tell me what was going on aside from the fact that she had bad abdominal pain.

I immediately jumped up and we went to see her at the hospital. She was doubled over in excruciating pain and couldn't even talk. The admitting ER doctor had called the GI surgeon to examine her. He had ordered a CAT scan and put her on a clear liquid diet. I went to the CAT scan with her and was terrified at what I saw. There was free air in the image; she had a perforated bowel, which meant that there was a hole in her intestines and she was leaking fecal matter into her abdomen.

Extremely alarmed, I pointed out the free air to the surgeon. This was a fatal situation! I told him she needed to go to the OR immediately. He disagreed with me. I was shocked. I could see on my mother's face that she was dying and things would soon get critical without immediate intervention.

I ducked out to call my nurse manager at Yale and explained the situation. She gave me Jeff's number and I told him what was going on. He asked if she was stable. She was, for now. He then asked to speak to the attending surgeon. Within minutes, an ambulance was waiting at the door. We loaded up and flew down the highway to Yale, where they basically rolled out the red carpet for my mother. She bypassed the ED and got into surgery immediately.

I saw Jeff for the last time as he scrubbed into surgery and I wished him Godspeed. His entire surgical team was there, and they operated for seven hours and removed numerous liters of infected abdominal fluid. My mother, still in critical condition, spent the night sedated in the SICU. Jeff's team would do an additional series of surgeries in the coming days as needed. Finally, my mother returned to the house. She was bedridden, with a series of fistulas and suction at the bedside.

My poor parents tried their best to navigate this near-lethal event, and the post-op recovery was not easy at all. The family's dynamic changed completely, as my mother could not get out of bed and my father had to tend to her around the clock. My brother, who was cognitively impaired, had previously been completely reliant on my mother for the most basic of needs. But somehow, her sickness had caused a spark of independence that neither I nor my father had ever seen before to ignite within him. He began doing things like making meals, doing dishes, taking the dog out, and taking care of his truck. It was very fascinating to see him blossom and spring into action when he needed to; his capabilities were actually much higher than any of us ever anticipated. As time went on, my mother had four additional surgeries, an ileostomy bag, and all of her reproductive organs removed.

I continued to live my life and work as a SICU nurse. I was suddenly a hero who had saved his mother from certain death and was pedestalized in my family's eyes. "Asher, you saved your mother's life." "Your family is so lucky to have you." As is a common theme throughout my life, I needed validation for everything I did, big or small, and I was receiving it. The act of saving my mother's life would come to save me in the future when I needed rehab but couldn't afford it. She decided to pay for my treatment out of her own money, as she saw it as a debt to be honored. I feel that it was fair; my last stint in rehab did end up saving my life, so I guess we're even. After saving my mother's life, she and I grew much closer until my addiction took over.

Throughout my life, the relationship between my mother and I was very...bipolar. Hot and cold, and sometimes explosive. No one in my family knew how and when to completely push my buttons like my mom. In hindsight, I can actually see that those "buttons" are usually sensitive areas within us that we need to expose and work on, but at the time it always just felt like a pointed attack. But a family dynamic is usually more complex than just mother and son, and mine was no exception.

The definition of survival is "the state or fact of continuing to live or exist, often despite difficulty or danger" (Oxford Dictionary). Everyone is just trying to live and is doing their best with what they've got, right? We're all dealt a different hand in life, and my brother Kevin is no exception. He was born with the cord wrapped around his neck, depriving him of oxygen. As he entered school, his teachers noticed a delay in cognition, and today, he's an eight-year-old child in a forty-year-old's body.

Adderall and Other False Prophets

Kevin received a lot of attention growing up, from teachers, aides, therapists, and especially my mother. From a young age, he was taught to depend on my parents for everything, even going to the bathroom. Now, at forty, he's tried to live on his own many times. He always ends up in a psychotic depression, usually resulting in an inpatient stay and loss of his apartment or condo.

Now, he doesn't *want* to be in a psychotic depression, and I guarantee he has no insight as to why it happens whenever he tries to move out. Even more interesting is the fact that my parents are also blind to the reason this happens every time (because they're part of the issue). After spending three months inpatient at any given psychological hospital, he ends up back at home living with them. My parents (especially my mother) then calm down and coddle him for a while, before waiting for enough time to pass to repeat the behavior. It's like an invisible never-ending loop they can't perceive.

I know why they do this: they aren't going to live forever, and the kid needs to have semi-independent living somewhere. And I certainly can't take him on in my present state, without home, income, or freedom. Everyone in this situation is just trying to live and survive the best way they know how, but they all keep hitting the wall of mental pathology.

This triangulated survival structure between my mother, brother, and father has been going on since my brother was born in 1985. My mother has been mired in guilt for Kevin's whole life due to the cord incident, even though it wasn't her fault. As soon as the diagnosis of cognitive impairment came, my parents went into lockdown mode to make sure he was covered every minute of every day. It was at this point that he became the identified patient, although neither he nor my parents knew it was happening (they were a young couple on their own without help from family and were taking care of themselves to the best of their ability). Kevin grew up learning that to survive, he had to rely completely on my parents, or else he'd have no chance (or so he believed). In my parents' eyes, nothing is ever good enough for Kevin and the world is always trying to fuck him over. Therapist after therapist has identified this, but it threatens the integrity of the triangle. Rejected, next provider please! He's up against a massive wall of learned helplessness. Sadly, they know not that they foster learned helplessness, it is just in their way of parenting.

When the brain faces something that it cannot logically find a solution or explanation for, it panics. If the stressor continues to press the person, this panic will advance to paranoia or delusional thinking, whatever the brain has to do to deal with the issue. Ultimately, it will confabulate reality if the stressor is chronic and severe enough (remember this, it will come up again later). My brother ended up in a delusional and psychotic state during the last time he tried to live outside of my parents' home. His literal mode of survival was threatened, and, when he yelped, my parents responded as they always have, bringing him home. No one wants this for him and, as bright as my parents are, I can't blame them for not seeing this for what it is, because it is antithetical to their mode of survival for Kevin. They truly believe they are helping when all they're doing is making him more and more dependent on them.

Ultimately, I will end up taking in my brother. Even though I know he could handle some level of independent living, I don't think it will ever be realized, and I'll eventually end up taking the role of my parents. It's just too much of a primal impulse; when his current mode of life is threatened, it creates massive mental pathology that lasts for quite some time, even with inpatient intervention. Kevin's entire life was engineered by my parents and now he is tasked with finding himself at age forty with cognitive impairment. This will be very difficult and his conditioning runs deep.

Saddlebrooke Annual Camping "Trip"

When I was in my twenties, I kept in great touch with all my guy friends from home. There were about a dozen of us, spread all over the Northeast, with some as far away as California and Florida. We were a tight group, always having each other's backs, from grade school straight through to adulthood. We were always getting in trouble together, making awesome memories at the same time. Stories from our respective bachelor parties alone could be their own book!

Adderall and Other False Prophets

Whenever we got together, things would get crazy. But a particular camping trip stands out in my mind as truly one for history books. The yearly camping trip was an S-Tizzy (Saddlebrooke) staple; it was the perfect excuse to get together year after year. We were all busy building our empires in life, with the majority beginning to practice medicine or law. Some of the guys were starting families. So, you'd think that, as a group, we would be smarter and make better decisions than what you are about to read. Nope. Every last one of us was still a mess at that point, despite being in our late twenties. Men will always be little boys at heart; we can try our best to appear mature and responsible, but we're all messy kids deep down. If there's a man out there who somehow truly became a mature adult, he certainly wasn't part of our group.

Every January, I would book our campsite in western Massachusetts as soon as available sites and dates for the year were posted. This was after I spent weeks hounding the boys through a group email thread trying to find a weekend that worked for everyone between our jobs, wives, and other commitments. It was like pulling teeth, but the frustration was always worth it and everyone always thanked me for putting everything together.

Our camping trip in 2010 was shaping up to be the best one yet; we were old enough and deep enough into our careers that we finally had real money to throw around. Airbnb was just becoming popular at the time (and one of the guys coming on the trip actually knew one of the founders), so I decided to check it out late one night while planning the trip. When I was just about to pass out for the night, my cursor drifted across the screen and landed on a listing that was absolutely perfect in every way: a massive two-story cabin with more than enough beds to fit all twelve of us, a lake nearby with boats we could use, a game room with every fun thing you can imagine, and a fully-stocked bar. Score! It was gorgeous, like something out of an architecture magazine, and right in the middle of a mountain range near our usual campsite. It was as if someone had engineered the perfect setting for our camping trip.

I woke Abbie up to show her what I had found, making sure to emphasize how affordable and "practical" it was. She agreed that it was perfect for us, so I went ahead and booked it for the weekend in August we all agreed upon. I couldn't wait.

Lockwood

This cabin would be the perfect setting for our annual weekend of debauchery. I sent the Airbnb on the email chain. With that crossed off the list, we could move onto the next order of business: party favors. We were adults now, which meant that we had enough money and time to refine our taste in drugs. Back then, my favorites were just weed, alcohol, and mushrooms. Same for the rest of the group, too. A couple of the guys had crossed over into messing around with cocaine more. No big deal, though.

In the months leading up to the trip, the email thread continued and it was evident the crew was down for a mushroom trip since we had a nice place to stay (as opposed to the tents we used in prior years). I made sure that my connection was able to supply us with a quarter pound. I wanted to make sure we had enough drugs for everyone and then some. A week before the trip, I made an excuse to slip out of the house and went to pick up the mushrooms. Abbie had no clue that we planned to trip on mushrooms; I promised I would keep it to booze and a little bit of weed, nothing else. Sure, it was bullshit, but I was prepared to do anything to get to this magical luxury cabin on the top of a mountain with nothing near it for miles and miles. It was going to be the time of our lives.

In the weeks prior to the campout, I could barely focus on anything else. I was excited for the trip every year, but this time, this palace I booked brought my anticipation to a whole new level. On the day of, I decided that I would leave early in the morning and stop to pick up Michael on the way there. We were the schemers of our group and I wanted to get to the cabin before anyone else that day. His wife gave us her blessing and smiled, knowing that we would be up to no good for at least the next 48 hours (she was a reformed party girl who used to go to raves, so she could make a very educated guess about what mischief we were trying to get into). After we left Michael's house, he had me stop in a parking lot about two miles away. He came back to the passenger seat a few minutes later with his contribution to our stash: a "micro dose" of mushrooms. I laughed, and off we went.

Pink Floyd and Radiohead filled the car as we drove through the mountains. Following GPS, I turned onto a private road that was unpaved, disheveled, and on a steep incline. This proved to be a little bit of a challenge for my C300 and Michael, fully tripping on mushrooms at this point, worried out loud that we might get stuck. I knew he had taken too much, but he'd always been able to handle himself. The road proved to be a nonissue, and we drove for a few more minutes before coming to a clearing. There was the beautiful lake, complete with canoes, from the Airbnb listing. According to the property owner, the lake was about halfway between the start of the road and the cabin. I couldn't remember the last time I was this excited.

The cabin came into view as we finally arrived. Michael and I were speechless as we stared at the gorgeous structure. I was still in shock that I found such a cool place, and now it finally felt real. Michael and I ditched the car and keyed into the cabin. The inside was even better, with a working hot tub and three fireplaces. It was a man's ultimate dream house, complete with an actual regulation beer pong table on the first floor. After our full walkthrough, we each claimed a bed (not that we'd be doing much sleeping). With that squared away, we decided to do a little exploring before everyone else showed up.

We decided to go check out the quarry, which had long since filled with water and turned into a lake. According to the owner, it hadn't been operational in over 75 years and was now just a spot where reckless teenagers and adrenaline junkies came to go cliff-diving. There were no real warning signs or supervision: just an 80-foot drop into 50 feet of water. Michael started freaking out the moment we got up there, so we scrapped the idea and went back to the cabin. I'll say this: 80 feet feels a hell of a lot higher when you're standing at the edge looking down.

While we were unloading the beer and food and settling into the cabin, Michael offered me some mushrooms. At the time, I had a very strict personal policy regarding hallucinogens: I'll only partake if everyone around me is on them too, and we need to be either around a fire or walking in the woods. Since we were planning to hang out inside the cabin until everyone else showed up, I passed on the mushrooms for now. Michael decided to eat some more, but I wasn't worried. He was one of those rare guys who was both deeply intelligent and completely grounded, so I figured the chances of him bugging out were slim. I, on the other hand, was nowhere near self-actualization at that point in my twenties. Even though I liked to think I'd already faced a few of my demons, the truth is, I had barely even come close to scratching the surface. Funny thing is, looking back, I think people like Michael could see the storm brewing in me a lot more clearly than I could at the time.

Suddenly, we heard a noise outside that could only be a car bottoming out on that final rocky hump that led to the cabin clearing. A few moments later, a car with the vanity plate BLIND X pulled up to the cabin and parked in front. I immediately recognized the plate and, sure enough, Mason and his crew piled out of the vehicle. I hadn't seen Mason in a minute. He and I grew up next door to each other and were close then, still are now. Our families even still hang out from time to time.

I opened the door and went outside to meet him. He gave me a big hug and I slapped hands with the guys who rode with him. I helped everyone unload the car and bring everything inside, taking special care with the booze and an ounce and a half of weed (this was before recreational legalization in the state, and that amount was *definitely* criminal).

Mason, Michael, and I had a long history, and the conversation picked up without missing a beat. After the cabin tour, we showed Mason the quarter pound of mushrooms, and his eyes lit up like the bowl already burning in his hand. As you can probably tell, neither I nor my friends typically wasted any time getting psychoactive substances into our systems. After passing the bowl around a few times, we figured we were all high enough and set the mushrooms aside for later. With some time left to kill before the rest of the guys arrived, Mason had a great idea: we should go fishing! He knew we both loved fishing, so he packed two poles and some bait for us. Sweet! The two of us grabbed the fishing gear and took off.

Mason and I walked down to the lake, about an 18-minute hike. On the way down, our friend Andrew drove past us, packed into his car with three other people. He sucked at driving, and got so excited when he saw us that he slammed his skid plate into a rock. It sounded like a bomb went off. He rolled down the window and started going on about how it wasn't his fault, just like he always did. We rolled our eyes and helped him back up, pointing him in the right direction to get to the cabin. He was stoned and coked up, his usual party combo. Every time he drove like that, he'd start seeing phantom cop cars everywhere, and we'd have to talk him down. Still, he wouldn't stop driving in that state, and the older we got, the more it concerned us.

Side note: if anyone in our crew was going to drive while totally twisted, it was me (and they'd all tell you the same). Everyone agreed The Lock was a better driver fucked up than sober, and yeah, it was somehow true. Even my straight-edge friends would admit it. There were very few days I couldn't handle my substances behind the wheel. Not something I'm proud of, but I had this mutant-like ability to stay between the lines and under the limit, even with chaos going on in my brain and all around me. Looking back, I realized that it probably had something to do with the constant hypomanic energy – just enough adrenaline to keep me awake, alert, and following the basic rules of the road.

Mason and I finally made it to the lake around 2:00 p.m. I know that because I looked down at my watch (we didn't bring our phones with us, for reasons I still can't explain). There were four canoes by the shore, flipped upside down so they wouldn't collect rain. We picked the red one, got on either end, and flipped it over. Almost immediately, I saw a snake strike at Mason's ankle and dart off into the bushes. The look on his face was pure panic. The situation was fucked; we were more than fifty miles from the nearest hospital.

I ran over and checked the bite. Two clean fang holes. I pulled out my knife and cut an X over the wound, then tried to flush it. Now, I'm a snake guy, so I knew that a decent percentage of strikes are dry bites. But Mason was already starting to feel warm and nauseous, which wasn't a good sign. I'd recognized the snake as a copperhead. Not lethal, but definitely the kind of thing that'll fuck up your weekend. Trying to keep him calm, I told Mason he was going to be fine and went to reach for my phone. Right – I left it at the cabin. So had he.

With no other choice, we started hobbling up the road (those eighteen minutes were some of the longest of my life). By the time we got to the cabin, Mason was very obviously sick, and Andrew called 911. It took a minute to explain where we were, but luckily we had a legal address to give to the dispatcher. Mason sat down, we iced the bite, and forced fluids on him to keep him hydrated. Now, keep in mind that we were still hallucination-level stoned, so the whole thing was pretty fucking intense for him. Honestly, it was for me too. Suddenly we heard a helicopter, getting closer. We all went outside and walked over to the clearing next to the cabin to investigate.

As soon as we saw the medical symbol on the bottom of the chopper, we collectively breathed a sigh of relief. I guess they'd figured trying to drive up into the mountains would be too much of a pain in the ass, so they sent air support (probably the best choice, given how much faster the chopper was). It landed, and they motioned for us to stay back. Two paramedics came over with a stretcher and loaded Mason on before immediately getting an IV started. I saw fear in his eyes, which was actually a good sign (much better than the alternative, unconsciousness).

The helicopter took off, and we all went inside, still shaken from what had just happened. We decided to do a round of shots for Mason and made a group decision not to fuck with the canoes again. So within the first six hours of the camping trip, one of the guys had to be airlifted out because of a poisonous snake bite. Surely all the crazy shit was behind us now, right?

By the time everyone in the group finally arrived at the cabin (and got filled in on the Mason situation), it was already getting late, so we decided to walk over to the cliff jump just to check it out. Michael decided to stay behind and get the campfire started. The plan seemed reasonable enough, and ten of us made the hike over.

"Holy shit," Andrew said, stepping out to the edge of the cliff once we arrived. We were all thinking the same thing. The drop somehow looked even bigger than it did earlier. Naturally, we started chucking rocks into the water to test the depth. We watched the rocks hang in the air for an absurdly long time, which only drove home how fucking high up we really were. Uneasy, we decided to head back to the cabin.

As we got closer, the smell of smoke hit first, then came the sound of crackling wood. We got back to the cabin to find Michael sitting in front of the perfect campfire, already halfway into a mushroom trip after munching on a few caps from the QP. The boys thought that was an insane amount of shrooms (which it was, to be fair), but it would definitely get the job done. None of us were trip veterans, and half the group still thought we'd be seeing little green men walking around. I'd brought a water bottle full of crushed Seroquel (a powerful sedative), just in case anyone's trip went sideways. I think most of us felt better knowing we had something, proven or not, within reach to pull the plug if things got too dark. This was going to be awesome.

With everyone finally there, we each grabbed a handful of fungus and started chewing, preparing to be on another planet in thirty minutes. Everyone was participating, we were outside in the woods, all my rules had been fulfilled. While we waited for the effects to kick in, we all sat around the fire, drinking and talking.

Before I explain what happened next, let me give a little background info on Andrew. He and I met when we were still in diapers and grew up together. We spent summers together at the local swim club, obsessively playing Magic: The Gathering. We even had our first beer together as teenagers (he promptly barfed about three sips in). Messing up his car by driving over a literal *rock* was actually very on-brand for him; Andrew was the guy who was somehow always tripping over shit or trying to mack on girls who were way out of his league. As an adult, he was that particular type of annoying dude who got really keyed up talking about politics if he was doing cocaine. He somehow ended up as a corporate lawyer, which was baffling to me (sure, he was definitely book smart, but the guy could not get out of his own way to save his life). Despite all of this, we all loved him anyway. Every crew needs an Andrew; without him, who would be the butt of all the jokes?

Everyone's mushroom trip kicked in at a different time, depending on whether they ate more stems or more caps. Legend has it that the more caps you eat, the more visuals you get. I mostly took stems and a few caps, because I was a bitch and still remembered the bad trip I had in college. Michael had been there for that too, but he had no fear. Since my metabolism was the fastest, my trip hit in about twenty minutes. I knew I was feeling the effects when everything and nothing became funny at the same time. I could see shapes in the flames in front of me, which I remember thinking was really cool. Soon I realized that Michael was tripping pretty hard, and so was Andrew.

At one point, Andrew got up to go piss in the woods, away from the fire, while the rest of us kept booming and having a great time. My mood was excellent, and I felt connected to my friends, some of whom I hadn't seen in a year. Time passed, and somewhere in the middle of a deep conversation, Michael asked where

Andrew was. That's when I realized he'd gone to piss like an hour ago. The thing about mushrooms is that time just stops existing. If you try to stare at a clock, it doesn't make any sense.

Great, now we had to stop everything to go track him down. Andrew was not a guy who could survive in the woods alone while sober, let alone on hallucinogens. We walked around the immediate area of the camp, yelling his name to no response. Fucking great. Someone got eaten by a bear. Let me tell you what it's like trying to form search parties with ten of your best friends who are all tripping balls: chaotic. We split into two teams and started combing the woods. Ten minutes turned into fifteen, into thirty, into forty-five. By that point, I was scared. Both search parties had made it back, but Andrew hadn't. I stood there staring up through the trees and caught a flash on the mountain next to us. It wasn't that high up, but I swear I saw what looked like a flashlight. Yeah, maybe I was seeing shit, but he had been gone long enough that I needed to do something.

Michael and I split off from the group, giving them a fake story about going to check the quarry again. In reality, we climbed that mountain. Maybe it was because of the mushrooms, but the climb took a lot less time than we expected. We walked the ridgeline of trees until we finally came across Andrew. He was lying on the ground, staring at the sky, flashlight still in his left hand. "Do you ever wonder what fucking pile of goop humans came from?" Very poetic, Andrew. Did you hear us calling for you? "No. The only noise I've heard was from the universe." While I was glad we found him and that he was clearly having a good time, part of me was pissed he'd just taken off like that. He and I had been Eagle Scouts and knew what to do, but the rest of the group didn't, especially not while tripping on mushrooms. Michael and I told him it was time to go back to camp as we helped pull him to his feet, laughing about the ridiculousness of the whole situation.

By the time we got back, the boys were deep into a serious game of beer pong. They'd drawn up a full tournament bracket and were already mid-round. Michael and I were just happy to see everyone together, laughing, high-fiving, letting loose, having a blast. That's what the campout was for. Even though we were grown, working, married, and living all over the place, we could still bring it back once a year and just be boys having fun.

Adderall and Other False Prophets

The next day, we all woke up at different times and started trickling into the cabin's many bathrooms, blowing each and every one up (an unfortunate side effect of the mushrooms). Michael was downstairs making bacon, eggs, and coffee, which we were all grateful for. After breakfast, we decided to walk back over to the quarry, this time in our bathing suits. I have to say, out of everyone, six guys jumped that year (which is an impressively solid number of guys willing to face the unknown). All we really knew was that the owner said people had done it before, but he wouldn't recommend it himself. That was enough of an endorsement for us. No matter how successful and responsible we looked to the outside world, we were the same crazy people we'd always been.

Somehow still high on mushrooms, Michael went first, staying in a perfect pencil shape as he entered the water. I went second, mostly because Michael had survived. I stepped up to the ledge and stared down at the greenish water below. Why did the drop seem to get higher each and every time we visited the quarry? I knew I couldn't overthink it, so I jumped straight down, careful not to launch out and accidentally add footage to the fall. *Ouch.* My right arm flew out from my body as I violently entered the water with a smack. I resurfaced with a nice black-and-blue bruise covering the inside of my arm.

Then came Andrew, doing his stupid WWE-style countdown before he jumped. True to form, he was completely off-balance. When he hit the water, it sounded like a firework going off. He'd basically done a belly flop, and his abdomen lit up bright red on impact. By the time we dried off and headed back to the cabin, he had a full black-and-blue bruise across most of his torso. I was pretty sure his internal organs were still intact, but I tried not to let on that I was vaguely concerned about the impact and shearing force.

In the end, we somehow all survived the weekend (even Mason), and the trip went down in history as our craziest one yet. Despite some of the scarier moments, the trip is a memory that I'll remember and treasure forever. And not because of the awesome cabin, or the tons of drugs. My friends were, and still are, family to me. They're the kind of real family that's nonjudgmental and always there with a warm greeting when I reach out. I knew they were always at arm's reach, and because of that, I felt safe instead of vulnerable.

Lockwood

My immediate family, on the other hand, hasn't always provided that same feeling. Over time, I've slowly grown to know and understand them, and today they're much more emotionally present and accessible – especially to my two boys. Kids see people exactly as they are – which is extremely anxiety-provoking for someone like me, who struggles so much with vulnerability – and for a long time, I didn't accept or love myself for who I actually was. It wasn't until I found some real self-acceptance that I could actually show up for them, and stay.

*   *   *

It's been a decade since the last campout. I fell into addiction and deeper into mental illness, and somewhere along the way, I lost touch with most everyone. Now, I am working on rebuilding those friendships and have the goal of perhaps one day bringing the camping trip back. Those people, and that time together, meant more to me than I ever said out loud.

Silver Hill Sorrow

Let me rewind a tiny bit back to when I moved in with Abbie while working at Yale. It was a bit of a change for me to deal with the transition from boyfriend to Abbie with our own place, to the two of us living together. This caused some depression symptoms and made themselves apparent, to which Abbie helped me the best she could. I eventually started getting panic attacks while on my shift in the SICU, so I eventually had to resign. I just couldn't cut it anymore. I moved back in with my parents, and Abbie moved back to her hometown in New York State. This lasted about six months before I followed her to live with her and her parents.

Living with her family was positive for my symptoms. The household was very tight-knit and her parents were steady support for us. This gave us a stable foundation to return to the world of academia in 2007 for graduate school, her as a nurse anesthetist and myself a psychiatric nurse practitioner. We had each other, her family, and school to keep us occupied. This stage of my life was very calm, but Teenage Asher still lived within me.

After graduating, we worked in our respective fields, which were very high-income. We bought a huge, beautiful house, too big for us at the time (but we could afford it). Between home improvement projects, traveling, friends, family, and our professional responsibilities, we stayed very busy and healthy.

This lasted until 2016. We still had it all: together for 16 years, married since 2009, German cars in the driveway, still proud owners of our dream house in her hometown. Both of us were successful in our careers...in fact, I had just opened a new psychiatric practice with multiple providers and about $80,000.00 worth of improvements. I should have been on top of the world.

A new addition to our life was coming: Giovanni, our soon-to-be-born son, whom we were lucky to conceive. However, Abbie's pregnancy had triggered unidentified fear within me. Teenage Asher inside me became terrified at the thought of the new responsibilities and change this would bring to our otherwise stable life. I began to implode, working longer and longer hours. I expanded my practice to house eight providers and a burgeoning wellness center. I had even gotten the idea for new telemedicine software, and investors were interested. I began forming a corporation.

I engaged in other forms of self-sabotage at the time, various drugs, short-lived affairs, partying with the boys, anything to take my mind off of the looming fear of fatherhood and responsibility. But my biggest thing was work. Fueled by Adderall, my drug of choice (originally obtained through a legitimate diagnosis of ADHD), I worked around the clock.

Adderall was great. I could stay awake longer, process more information, have a competitive mental edge, and handle all my responsibilities. It seemed to help me balance it all: running my practice, the wellness center, my home life, and starting my tech company. Soon, I began eschewing things like sleep, nutrition, hydration, sanity, my family, and myself in favor of pills and work. The amphetamines were uncontrollably fueling the manic side of my bipolar and I was soon experiencing things like hypersexuality, irritability, aggression, and delusions of grandeur. I was impulsive, and the mania made me unable to make properly informed decisions. Sometimes, I was awake for days, and keeping such odd hours has a way of attracting seedy individuals who seem to only come out at night. My circle expanded to some less-than-desirable company.

I grew more distant from Abbie as her pregnancy progressed. Suddenly, her delivery date was here. I managed the day she gave birth absolutely fine but immediately became absent the next day as my life flew off the tracks. I was having a full-blown affair with a colleague and was fully addicted to Adderall at this point. This led to massive sleep deprivation, which caused my bipolarity to crack with raging symptoms. I was running from responsibility and myself, and I was suddenly on full tilt, fueled by drug addiction, money, cars, strippers, and cocaine. I sought out anything that would distract me and produce dopamine, as I didn't think I could be a good father. I just wasn't good enough.

As I became unpredictable, Abbie wanted nothing to do with me and she realized she needed to protect newborn Giovanni. One of the last times I saw him before she left me, he was in his car seat in the master bedroom. I had been awake for days on Adderall and could barely keep my eyes open. I was lying next to him, his hand in mine, both of us passed out. When I woke up, it was nighttime and the house was empty. Abbie had left with Giovanni. I was still lying on the floor in the same position. I had never felt more alone than at that moment.

I didn't let that feeling stop me; I began to spend even more time at my office and with Vlad, my business partner for my new tech corporation. We frequented local strip clubs, of which I had my favorites. Cocaine was a useful currency at these clubs since the girls had to be up all-night dancing, it was a natural match. At this point, I was doing about 500-600 mg of Adderall a day (the FDA maximum is 60 mg). Unfortunately, in addition to wakefulness, another side effect is appetite suppressant. I was losing weight, continuing to not sleep, and my mental illness was raging. I needed to get some help and have some time for myself. I decided in January 2017 to enter a 30-day inpatient rehab program at Silver Hill in New Canaan, Connecticut.

Silver Hill was backed by Yale and was a beautiful establishment. My aunt drove me there from Upstate New York, my head bouncing off the dashboard from exhaustion. I entered the rehab hot. I told the admitting physician to go fuck himself, that I was a medical professional and knew what was best for me. Great start.

I slept for two days straight in detox, sleeping so deeply that they were able to draw blood without waking me. When I finally woke up, I had never been so hungry in my whole life, with a thirst equally as vicious. I devoured everything in the snack area, including sugar packets. This was the first time I experienced full withdrawal from Adderall. I regained composure and became aware that I was sharing my room with someone else in detox.

Trent was from Nebraska, part of a rich real estate family who owned something like 2% of the land in the state. He was there to kick dope, much harder than Adderall (but equally as dangerous). Despite the uncomfortable physical symptoms he was experiencing as he detoxed, he was able to keep me engaged in conversation when I was conscious. Soon, we were both able to stand up straight and talk without issue, and we were moved to the boy's house, where we roomed together.

In general population, we had a campus meeting at the center hall with both the boys and girls. It was there I first met Melissa. Melissa was this cute little blonde who had become hooked on opiates after multiple back surgeries. She had lost her husband to suicide and I decided she needed to be rescued (I was wrong). In rehab, I would end up trading addictions, Adderall for Melissa. Oh yeah, as an aside: never get a girlfriend in rehab.

I originally decided to enter rehab just to take a break from all the action in my life, and it seemed to be working so far. I began gaining back all the weight I had lost on Adderall. The food at Silver Hill was incredible. It was a buffet, set up with stations like a wedding. After eating, everyone was allowed to take a smoke break back behind the building before heading back to their dorms. One night, I was about to get on the bus back to the boy's house when Melissa asked me to have a smoke with her. I locked eyes with one of the senior guys, who gave me a look of judgment that said, "you are choosing a new addiction over your recovery". I knew exactly what he was trying to get across, but I went with her to enjoy that cigarette anyway. It was this excursion that ignited the cross-addiction; Adderall was fully gone from my system and I needed something to fill the void. Melissa did as well and it appeared her and I were on the same page.

Even though my psychologist at the time had given me a packet on cross-addiction, I was far from recognizing it in myself. I was just replacing one addiction with another; Melissa was able to cause a rise in dopamine in my neural reward center that felt equal to or larger than the one caused by Adderall. Before I knew it, I was buying presents off Amazon and having them delivered to her dorm in the girl's house. I was sending her so many things daily that Amazon packages got banned on campus. I didn't realize that I had actually entered a hypomanic state, fueled by the relationship instead of exogenous chemicals.

Things that are not chemicals can trigger emotional episodes that mirror the effects of drugs. In this instance, my brain was looking for a reward because I was no longer giving it drugs, so it zeroed in on Melissa. She was in the same boat; without opiates, she was looking to fill her dopamine void with something rewarding, too. We were becoming addicted to each other. Whenever I saw her on campus, a warm, euphoric feeling would spread through my body, filling the dopamine void. The speed with which our relationship grew was pathological at best. She ended up becoming my sole focus at Silver Hill because I needed to replace the dopamine spike of Adderall with *something*. If she hadn't been there, I would have just found something or someone else to hyperfocus on.

On Family Weekend, my parents and brother showed up, along with Abbie and my aunt. I wasn't looking forward to this weekend; I knew my family could see right through me and I wasn't putting in the work. This was the first time I had seen my wife and Giovanni in a long time, and they bumped into Melissa in the center hall. That wasn't terrible, but my counselors did stage an intervention during a group activity that set off my anger (which can be extreme during a hypomanic episode). I was hooked on the dopamine spike from my addiction to Melissa, and since she wasn't there during this exercise, I was irritable and impulsive.

Family Weekend culminated in a discussion with Abbie regarding the tech corporation I had founded. By this point, we had just received a quarter of a million dollars in seed funding. She wanted me to end it, but I wasn't willing to give up on my multi-million-dollar idea. Abbie said something about Vlad that triggered an impulsive episode. It was at that moment that I traded my wife and son for bullshit. I stormed out of the family event and threw my wedding ring into the abyss outside. I didn't fully comprehend the consequences in the heat of the moment, but that event marked the end of my 16-year relationship with one of the best people I have ever known. I ran back across campus to my dorm, feeling excruciating pain and exhaustion like I never had before. I felt dark and alone and it hit me that my time with Abbie was over.

That night, after everyone had left, I went into the bathroom in the dorm. I saw a ladybug on the rim of the sink. I thought this was strange but didn't pay much attention as I got into the shower and slid the door shut. I needed to decompress from everything that had just happened. Halfway through the shower, I suddenly became violently ill and began vomiting. I continued to vomit every 15 minutes for the next 12 hours and was in absolute searing pain. I was lying on the floor of that marbled bathroom, waiting for death. Was I transcending out of my 16-year codependent relationship and taking control over my life again?

When I woke up the following day feeling completely debilitated, I pulled myself upright and saw the same ladybug on the rim of the sink. It had survived, and so had I. I've long believed that our thoughts and emotions play out not only in the mind but also physically. The 12-hour breakdown of my physical body was the severing of true love, but I didn't connect the dots at the time.

The last two weeks of rehab were spent courting Melissa and completely ignoring the healing process, AA meetings, therapy, classes, etc. We became quite the couple on campus and amassed an entourage of followers, as we were the closest model of a "normal" relationship anywhere in this biodome. During my last week, I met with Dr. Schneider to be processed out of rehab. I'll never forget what she told me: "This is your only chance to regain your life, status, family, everything." I ignored her. What did she, a renowned physician of 35 years, know over my personal and medical knowledge? According to me, she was ignorant. She saw how far I was off the path of my life and called it like it was. I tried to call her bluff, incorrectly, and ran in the opposite direction. In reality, I knew she was right.

By this time in the house, I was a senior and was very popular amongst the guys because I represented everything they could no longer touch or have. In a way, I was the artificial dopamine spike that they needed, but caution was heeded. The guys who ran the boy's dorm made sure I wasn't too much of a "leader" in the eyes of my peers, but I didn't mind (my mind was on Melissa). I was entirely disinterested in healing and sobriety and it was obvious. Part of me felt bad as I knew the new guys were looking up to me, but I was too addicted to her to care about much else. Every second of every day my mind was entirely focused on Melissa. My biggest hurdle before my discharge was that I still hadn't been able to be physical with her due to the rules on campus. It became my goal to hook up with her. So far, all we had been able to do was sneak into a handicapped bathroom stall and make out.

My original discharge date was supposed to be Monday, February 20, 2017. I was able to negotiate release on Sunday, the 19th. Perhaps this request changed the course of my life forever, maybe not. That day, Vlad rolled up in a car filled with balloons to pick me up. I ran from my house into the smoking area outside and grabbed Melissa, making out with her in full view of everyone on campus. I didn't care about rules anymore, I was about to bounce! I was scolded one last time as I gathered my things inside and said my goodbyes but I barely noticed. I was free! I had graduated, I did it and no one could take it away from me. I had "beat" addiction in my 30-day residential inpatient rehab, conveniently hidden out of New York State as a private program.

I let go of the balloons out the window and we peeled out of the campus parking lot, flying back to New York. The second we were on the road, I remember feeling the urge for Adderall returning, and I didn't know why. Now, it's obvious that the dopamine spike from spending time with Melissa was gone, and that void needed to be filled (we had exchanged cell numbers and she had given me access to her Facebook so we could link up on the outside, but for now, she was still stuck at Silver Hill for another 5 days). I think I was actually hungrier for a spontaneous relationship than I was for drugs, but really, anything would do.

Once back home, my business partner brought me up to speed on what had happened at the practice while I was gone. I was immediately swamped with work, and that wasn't even counting the ensuing divorce and the sale of our beautiful house. I jumped back in headfirst and started using again the day I got out of rehab. With so much work to be done, I needed to up the ante a little bit: I started snorting lines of what we called "Freud's Dynamite": crushed Adderall mixed with levomilnacipran, a SNRI that targets adrenaline. I was off to the races. I became so focused on drug use, my practice, and the new corporation that I didn't even have time to think about how I had fucked up my beautiful life and destroyed it in the blink of an eye.

After the failed rehab stint, more drug use, and continued erratic behavior, Teenage Asher finally had what he wanted: no responsibilities and a life filled with constant pure dopamine spikes. Abbie was destroyed while I bathed in the filth of my horrible decisions. There was just so much I couldn't deal with that aborting the marriage seemed like my only option. The bipolar nineteen-year-old within me couldn't handle the thought of becoming second in line to her after the baby's arrival, just like I had always been second in importance to my parents after my brother. There was no way I could have handled fatherhood at that time.

We divorced, and Abbie continued picking up the pieces of the life that used to be ours. She bought a new house, took care of Giovanni, and continued her job at the hospital. She eventually began a relationship with a man you can describe as "safe". Meanwhile, I continued my rampage of destructive behaviors.

Self-Righteous Suicide

Two days after returning home from rehab, Vlad dragged me out of my office, insisting I needed a break. I really didn't feel like going out; I was heavily focused on work and the news that Melissa would be discharged from Silver Hill in a couple of days and would be returning to her home in Connecticut. Regardless, we ended up at one of my favorite nearby strip clubs. I spent the first part of the night distracted. Melissa kept calling me and each time I needed to run outside so she didn't hear the music in the club.

In between calls, I ran into Aileen, one of the dancers at the club. I still remember vividly the moment she turned the corner, pushing Vlad out of the way to focus entirely on me. We shook hands in front of the owner of the club and I bought her a drink. Aileen and I ended up talking for four hours that night. The conversation felt so natural and fluid, it was as if we had known each other for years (or maybe it just felt that way because my dopamine void wasn't getting filled by Melissa or drugs at that moment). Aileen, too, had addiction problems and was at the end of a bad marriage. I was her new dopamine spike and she was mine. I sent Vlad home in an Uber and took Aileen back to the hotel I was staying at since I had been kicked out of my house.

Back at the hotel, we partied hard. We both had cocaine, weed, and booze. I had a full script of Adderall on me, so we were awake all night and into the next day. The sex was great (everyone is right, the crazy girls know what they're doing in bed). When morning came, I dropped her off at her car and immediately sped to Vlad's house to share the news about my exciting night. He was in bed, asleep. I jumped right in and started giving him a play-by-play of everything that had happened since we parted ways the night before.

Once again, I was running from myself as I swiftly traded one addiction for another, over and over again and in a severe manic state. In three days time, I went from Adderall to Melissa to Aileen and then back to Adderall. But I wasn't totally finished with Melissa yet; we met up at a hotel in New Haven on the day of her release (I told Aileen I was going to be visiting my family). Melissa had already relapsed too, so partying wasn't a problem. I got to finally have my way with her, and she left claw marks down my back to prove it. After that, I didn't want to hang around too long. Melissa's recent ex-boyfriend was an active member of the Russian mob, and I was eager to get back to the new girl who crowned my interest, Aileen. I never saw Melissa again after that. I'm pretty sure the ex found out about our rendezvous and put her in the hospital over it. I had my new source of dopamine, anyway.

On the way back to New York from visiting Melissa, I fell asleep on the drive. Still fucked up from partying, I rolled my car two times, landed on my tires off the highway, and had a piece of metal sticking in my head. Both the mirrors had been ripped off my car and the roof was caved in. Everything was fuzzy when the trooper asked me if I knew where I was and if I had been drinking (I had). I managed to work into the conversation that I was a nurse practitioner. It was because of this that they decided to go easy on me and spare me a DUI or DWI. I ended up with fifteen tickets and spent the better part of eight hours in a local ER. Once again, I escaped from a bad situation due to my status and smooth talking. Vlad picked me up from the hospital and life continued for me in a blind manic state. I knew a local DA and called in the favor and got off of everything for $125.00 fine. Go figure. It's really who you know.

*   *   *

My soon-to-be ex-wife tried to warn me about Aileen, but I ignored her. Despite how nasty I had been to Abbie; she still took the time to call me one night and express the concerns she had about the dark energy around Aileen. She would end up being absolutely correct, but I laughed off her words of caution. She told me that Aileen would try to get knocked up. Aileen was my new source of dopamine and self-fulfillment, and *that* was what I couldn't ignore. For all I knew, Abbie could simply want to take my new source of happiness because she was bitter that I had left her and Giovanni. Drugs and illness and mania ruled every single thought process I had (barring clinical decision-making, which had somehow remained intact).

Lockwood

It eventually became time for Abbie and I to clean out the home we once shared in preparation for the imminent sale. I saw a picture of the three of us, Abbie, Giovanni, and myself, and it set me off emotionally. I was immediately shifted back to reality, and an overwhelming feeling of failure and shame came over me. As I ruminated over all I had lost and what had become of the family I started, I lost it (and I mean *big time* lost it). I pulled a large bottle of Xanax and a bottle of gin from my belongings and left the property with the intent to end my life.

After I left, Abbie called the state police to report me as suicidal. I drove my Mercedes C300 to a secluded empty parking lot, far away from any main roads. I washed down handful after handful of pills with gin. My head began to fog as I could hear four counties' worth of police sirens, swarming any area where I might possibly be.

They didn't find me, and I began to lose my vision as the drugs took hold. My brain felt like Jello as I somehow focused on a recent thought: one of my great friends, Dr. Cohen (a locally famous OBGYN), had told me to text him if shit was ever going down and I was in trouble. If there was ever a time when I was in trouble, this was it. The message reached him. I still don't know how he did it, but he scrubbed out of surgery upon receiving my SOS. He flew down the highway in his Audi R8 to where I was hiding with my pills and alcohol. He somehow got me on my feet and cleaned up my car a little.

I left with him in his car, and he found ways to keep me awake in the passenger seat as we passed squads of state and local law enforcement on the main roads in town. He drove me around for hours, keeping me awake to try and sober me up from all the drugs I had taken. Eventually, his beeper alerted him to an emergency surgery he needed to return to the hospital. Dr. Cohen drove me to Vlad's house, instructing him to keep me awake for as long as possible. I was still shrouded in a haze and barely remember being at Vlad's house.

Seeing the state I was in, and having no medical training, Vlad panicked and called the authorities. They were still out looking for me, and two officers soon showed up to Vlad's house. I stepped out calmly with them to head to the ER. Despite never having shown any religious proclivities in the past, Vlad left me with these parting words: "Jesus will watch over you," which I thought was odd, but I appreciated the sentiment, nonetheless.

When we got to the ER, I was still fully inebriated by benzodiazepines and alcohol. I suddenly became enraged and combative, refusing to get on a stretcher. An orderly barked at me to get on the bed or he would do it for me. I was all of 142 pounds at this point, and this guy was massive. I started to mouth off to him and he suddenly slammed me on the stretcher, a man of his word. I recognized some of the staff swirling around me, and I'm sure they recognized me, a renowned local private-sector psychiatric nurse practitioner with a huge practice and thousands of patients under his belt. It must have been sad for them to see one of their own in such a state, but at the moment, I continued being an asshole and didn't deserve any of the courtesy they would show to me. They knew that the decision to take one's life comes in stages, and I hadn't been able to bring myself to complete the final stage: ultimately, I wanted to live.

The admitting psychiatrists made the merciful decision to hide me on a medical floor rather than the psych unit. My stay in the inpatient locked ward would have only highlighted my visit to the hospital and the struggles I was having. Hours into my stay, I was still rude and cocky, giving only smart-ass answers and being a jerk to everyone. I wasn't the Asher I had known for 35 years. Eventually, the team decided to send me downstate to get off the benzos, to a truly locked asylum called the Westchester Institute.

They sent me there at night, suffering the entire 40-minute highway ride by myself in an ambulance. Upon arrival, all I could see was the massive dark silhouette of the facility against the night sky. Immediately, I knew this would be much different than my stay at Silver Hill. I unceremoniously entered the building through a metal detector and security checkpoint before being led to a locked padded room with a security camera in the upper corner. A genuine locked padded room. I took this moment to ponder my situation. Before I was on top of the world, and now I felt like nothing more than a spectacle to the general public. I was on a self-destruct mission and couldn't get out of my own way. I needed help, but I had pushed away everyone good in my life. I was sick but still very capable at this point.

Lockwood

Sitting in the padded room, I started to withdraw hard from the Xanax. I developed shakes as my blood pressure spiked. I was left alone in that state for about an hour and a half before the admitting psychiatrist came in to do my intake. After the interview, I was brought up to 4 West, a legendary locked ward for the "criminally insane" and those with severe mental illness. I was brought to a room with two other guys and not enough beds (evidently, I was to sleep on the floor). One of my roommates was in for psychosis and sexual assault and the other was in for treatment-resistant schizophrenia. I was certainly in with the sickest of the sick; maybe this was where I really needed to be.

Despite all this, Westchester was actually a good institution with a long history in the psych community. I was placed here to be hidden away from the public eye while I obtained treatment. I wasn't in a place to appreciate it at the time, as my relationship with Aileen was blossoming and it was hard to be away from her for an indeterminate amount of time. The attending physician on my unit, Dr. Singha, saw me that morning and he had me pegged. He noted initially that once my detox from benzos was over, I would be discharged. This was exactly what I wanted to hear. The goalposts were in place and soon I would return to my beloved. Only one thing stood in my way: Darcy, my social worker. She stated that I should stay for three to six months in order to fully stabilize and get away from any potential bad relationships. My parents agreed with her. I fully opposed her, naturally, and maneuvered to get discharged by Dr. Singha. Even though Darcy had been completely correct, I was manic and capable and had a way with words. I detoxed and talked my way out of that ward.

Aileen was my main source of dopamine, and she reciprocated, making it even better. My brain would do whatever it took to get this hit, because that's how it is for an addict. I lived for dopamine hits, day to day and week to week. The inner voice telling me this was a bad idea was completely obliterated by addiction and mental illness. I needed a steady flow of good feelings to try and pull me out of the hole of depression I had fallen into, and Aileen and Adderall were perfect for that. Planning and thinking had completely fallen to the wayside.

As I got used to Westchester, Aileen made it a point to call the payphones we had access to as much as possible. She called so frequently that my buddies on the unit would have to pick up the phone for me when I wasn't available. At this point, I was completely out of my mind, focused only on the singular goal of getting discharged as soon as possible to be with her. More specifically, the sex was incredible, so I had a drive to repeat that behavior over and over. Basic actions like food, sleep, whatever, produced a dopamine spike something like twice the baseline. Cocaine is four times that, Adderall ten times that, but being with her felt like a hundred times baseline.

Sleeping and thinking became a problem as I was on a 10-day trajectory to come off of maximum-dose Xanax. It felt like the two hemispheres of my brain were rotating in opposite directions, which is something I wouldn't wish on anyone. To lessen the withdrawal and keep me medically safe, I was given low-dose Klonopin and Gabapentin. Having Aileen to talk to every day really helped the tapering process. Some of my good friends came to visit me, people who would end up gradually dropping out of my life in the coming years (who wants to associate with drug addicts who abandoned their family for affairs and pharmaceuticals?). I spent my 35th birthday within those walls, and every now and then I would ponder how I let my life get to this point.

Eventually, I felt it was time for my stay at Westchester to come to an end. I made sure I was completely tapered off the Xanax. Dr. Singha and his entourage of doctors felt I was medically cleared to leave, but Darcy disagreed. She shared her thoughts with my parents, which led to me staying a little longer than I had hoped. This wasn't all bad, though, because it forced me to engage with the other patients more. Entering the facility, I was high and mighty and saw myself as "above" everyone else who was locked up there. As I got to know them more, I found myself in surprisingly enriching conversations with those who had nothing to their name. Some of the talks I had with those guys were better than those I had with any friends or colleagues outside. I'll never forget Donnie, a fifty-five-year-old drunk bipolar man who talked with me at length about what's really important in life. I can still see in my mind the $1 Monopoly bill where he wrote his phone number and the message "*Never blow off your kid. Call me.*" Although I wasn't yet ready to heed his message, it was the best advice anyone could have given me at the time. But parenting, providing, and communicating were not high on my hierarchy of importance as I was still searching for that next dopamine hit.

Finally, the day of my release came as Aileen arrived to pick me up. With the Xanax no longer clouding my brain, she actually looked a little bit different to me in a way I couldn't put my finger on at the time. In fact, my entire perception of reality had changed completely without the fog of heavy benzodiazepines shutting off my fear center. I had been on six milligrams of Xanax daily for 12 years, so the dulling of fear and anxiety had become my reality. Unfortunately, my new version of reality did not sense the true dangers of what, or who, was around me, either. People around me who knew and cared about me could sense it, but I was totally blind.

It feels important to mention that one of my congenital faults is that I am sometimes not immediately able to identify individuals as dangerous, which affords them time to get close to me and gain my trust. This was heightened by the combination of reduced fear from the Xanax and increased confidence from the Adderall. I wasn't in touch with my true reality and I was making decisions accordingly. Once they're in and have gained my trust, I'm blind. People with borderline personality disorder or narcissistic/sociopath traits especially seek this out in a potential victim. Anyone can put on a show and hide their true intentions for six months, and by then, they're completely ingrained in your life. As someone who was very dependent on outside variables for validation, as I've already mentioned, I was especially susceptible to this kind of outside manipulation. Due to my drug use, I was frequently in contact with seedy people. Once my relationship with them was established, they could get me to do things I wouldn't have otherwise done, like write them scripts. Dependency on anything external is a core weakness.

Anyway, I was very excited to see Aileen, new perspective or not. We got in her car and began heading north, back towards home . On the drive, Vlad called me to see how I was doing. He let me know that due to my suicide attempt, my entire practice (all eight providers and myself) were being evicted as of June 1, 2017. I found this ridiculous and headed to the office as soon as I was back home.

Silicon & Serotonin

Faced with the bad news, I immediately started planning my next move and how I would find a new space for myself and the other providers. A knock at the door alerted me to visitors, who turned out to be two goons the property owner had sent over. They escorted me to the main office building for a meeting with the owner's attorney. I was brought to a cement room containing nothing but a big table, some chairs, and a hanging light. There I sat with the two of them staring at me waiting for her arrival.

Following the theme, the lawyer began grilling me about what had happened when I OD'd on Xanax. Evidently, the police had stormed the office building while on their search for me. Since this had happened on a Sunday, the building had been empty except for one innocent worker trying to get a jump on the coming week. I learned that the police had basically pistol-whipped the guy when he exited a bathroom, thinking it was me. It was then that I learned that Abbie's police report had been misconstrued; the police asked her if I had access to any weapons, and she told them she didn't know but I had a shotgun locked up in storage that I hadn't used in years. This led to me being considered armed and dangerous and the poor man in the office building ending up in the hospital with his face rearranged. So I guess the owner was facing some legal ramifications, maybe, I wasn't sure. What I did know is that I should have had an attorney present since I was questioned by one. They knew that, too.

Days passed since the "interrogation," and I retained counsel for myself. The lawyers went back and forth and came to a compromise: the property manager would wash his hands of my ten-year, million-dollar lease if my practice and I went quietly. Unbeknownst to me, he had lost a brother to suicide, which made him sympathetic to my struggles. Had I not gone inpatient, he probably would have treated me a little harsher, but looking back, I respect it. At this point, I still thought I had all my skeletons safely locked up in a closet, but everyone knew what was going on.

Things were still humming along in the background with my telehealth corporation, and after closing things out with my practice, Vlad arrived with news.

Since we were fully seeded with funding and things were going so well, it was highly recommended that we take things to California, Silicon Valley, for further progress and development. A fork in the road was in front of me, and I had to make a decision. Should I leave everything behind me, including my newborn son, and forge ahead in Silicon Valley? At this point, it seemed to me as if Rome were burning and departure was inevitable. The decision felt natural to me, California seemed to offer the new beginning I needed as I continued to run from myself and my apparent issues.

I decided to completely shut down my physical practice in New York and continue it virtually from the West Coast while working on the corporation, Synaptic Link Telehealth Inc.

I took Aileen out to lunch to break the news to her, sure this would be the end of our growing relationship. She had three young kids to take care of and was still married to her soon-to-be ex-husband. Sitting across from her at a restaurant table, her response shocked me: "I'll go with you". This wasn't what I expected, but I went with it. She was all in, and I took this as a good sign. I excitedly told Jane, a long term friend and mentor. Jane warned against this decision, but I didn't listen. I couldn't understand why she wasn't happy for me.

*　　　*　　　*

We arrived at our eight-million dollar "tear down" mansion in Portola Valley, California, just outside of San Francisco. We had just received another quarter million dollars in seed money. The house was beautiful, on the side of a mountain facing Tech Valley. Aileen's three kids took off in opposite directions to claim their new bedrooms. Vlad took the guest house on the property. We had arrived on one of the hottest days on record, 115 degrees, and the air conditioning wasn't working in the house yet. We slept on the floors that night as our furniture and cars hadn't arrived yet. It felt like a brand-new chapter opening in my life, on that September 2, 2017. Endless possibilities unfurled before me, just waiting for me to grab them. I tried to push the words of a patient out of my head: "Asher, wherever you go, there you are." Everything felt new and fresh, and I didn't want to believe that all my problems from the East Coast, all of the addiction, mental illness, everything, had followed me here, too.

On our first full day in Palo Alto, we decided to visit a farmers' market. The heat was still blazing, the mansion was stuffy and we needed some fresh air. The six of us, myself, Aileen, the kids, and Vlad, piled into a car and off we went. On the road, it seemed like every car was a Tesla, and I noted the absence of bumper stickers and political statements. Everyone here was either a millionaire or homeless; there was no middle class. I was happy to be on the privileged side, despite the fact that I had much less liquid capital than any of my neighbors. I quickly learned that this wouldn't be obvious to the locals, as the standard uniform for billionaires tends towards ripped t-shirts, flip-flops, and a car worth less than $50,000.00. It was almost hard to tell who was who. Everyone here was accepting, and we never felt like outsiders.

At the farmers' market, we were astonished at how fresh and beautiful all the produce was, and it was all local. Despite being exhausted from our travels and sleeping on the floor, we marveled at the offerings as we traveled from booth to booth. Something crazy happened to me that day, and I still can't believe it. While traversing the market, my shoe caught on something and I stumbled to the pavement. Steadying myself, I looked to see the thing I tripped over was a person, sitting with a child in front of a street performer, none other than the founder of the largest social media site ever. Yes, that one. He stared back at me with his slate-colored t-shirt, bowl haircut, and complete lack of emotional tone. I opened my mouth to apologize but nothing came out, I was choking. He looked at me and said blankly, "You guys aren't from around here." Was it that obvious? Sure, we were wearing winter clothing, pale, visibly exhausted, and photographing everything. We were obvious transplants.

"We're here from New York, for a startup called Synaptic Link Telehealth. We just got in last night, but we're staying in Portola Valley." I introduced myself, Aileen, and Vlad. He asked what space our startup was in. I explained that we were in the interdisciplinary healthcare space looking to virtually connect primary care and mental health providers. Miraculously, he seemed interested in our little endeavor and invited us to lunch with him and his number two later that day. I couldn't believe our luck! Our first day in California and we were already making connections like this.

We immediately returned to the mansion to get ready for our priceless meeting later in the day. Aileen decided to take the kids to the zoo, leaving Vlad and I to prepare. We were to meet him at a sushi restaurant in downtown Palo Alto at 1:00 p.m.. We did our best to get cleaned up, as our luggage had still not been delivered by the movers. We left at 12:30 p.m. and got into an accident while merging onto the highway. I fully understood the strange new world we were in when the officer arrived and I didn't need to explain a thing to him, as a traffic drone had captured the entire scene.

Unfortunately, the presence of the drone did not speed up the process of recording the accident. Vlad and I ended up missing our lunch meeting that day. We hadn't gotten his cell phone number or personal email, so we weren't able to reach out to him to let him know what happened or reschedule. We told our software engineers what had happened, and they insisted it was good luck for our company. While I didn't see it that way, I still let the happenstance meeting fuel my grandiose perception of myself. I ran with it, thinking I was a god. It's worth mentioning that when I stumbled over him at the farmer's market, I was high as a kite. He probably recognized my Adderall-fogged look; we were all on it at that point, just to stay awake.

In California, my addiction to Adderall was in full control. I would stay up for days, virtually running my psych practice with my patients from back in New York, in addition to acting as CEO for the corporation. Friends I trusted back in New York were taking care of me on that front, as well as the ten prescriptions I needed to control my bipolar disorder. It was extremely hard to even get on a waitlist for a psychiatrist in California, let alone to get stimulants there. I was irritable and mean to Aileen, her children, and my soon-to-be ex-wife. Aileen seemed to relish in the drama I would cause, especially in my sleep-deprived state. She seemed to thrive in chaos, situations most people would pull back from. This should have been a red flag to me, but I paid no heed at the time. We fought constantly, and I identified her as the source of disturbance in the house. I began to project all my problems on her, seeing myself as the righteous light and her the instigator. This, combined with how big my ego had gotten due to my living in a mansion, gaining large capital investments, arranging meetings with bigwigs in the tech space, and my role as a medical provider and CEO, pushed me further into mania and drug addiction. I faced no consequences and nothing was going to stop me, short of calamity.

This would come soon enough, as our seed fund pulled the rest of her investment in November when she could see the struggles we were having on a personal level. This put me in a terrible position: as CEO, I had to maintain consistent monetary flow to the business. We were still about $150,000.00 short of the funds needed for software development. I needed to procure this quickly because the entire reason we were in Silicon Valley in the first place was to produce a functional product. I found a shady company that would leverage my personal credit to obtain ten lines of credit with obscenely large limits. I agreed without thinking, and this was the last time I would see a credit score above 700. I didn't question how the company did this; in my mind, I was a king, so of course I deserved access to that capital.

With cash flowing through the company again, our development team overseas resumed work on the software. We met with them regularly, and I was frequently approving cash advances of over $15,000.00 every couple of weeks. In the meantime, my personal virtual psych practice was grossing about $8,000.00-10,000.00 a month. Our rent at the mansion was $7,500.00 a month, so this worked for the time being. We began to pitch the software at various tech and health entrepreneur gatherings, like Health 2.0 in San Jose.

This was my first pitch in front of serious investors, but I quickly got used to it. I had practiced my slides and was wearing a full suit. With Vlad recording the event on his cell phone for YouTube, I absolutely crushed it. Soon I was swarming with fans, tech guys, and millionaires, waving around their business cards to set up meetings. My ego and addicted brain latched onto this dopamine hit and, instead of sitting with the satisfaction of a job well done, I sought out more of the same. I had always wanted to look important and be wanted by others, and this was the perfect venue.

In the moment, it felt like all this external approval was filling the void in me from childhood. The validation I wanted from my parents my whole life, which

I had tried to attain through sports and academics but was always just out of reach due to them being preoccupied with my brother, now seemed attainable. In New York, I had built a medical practice that rivaled those in Manhattan, and still nothing from them. I had taken cognitive enhancers and imploded my marriage while trying to grab the brass ring, but they still hadn't reached out to me to make sure I was okay like they would my brother. I continued to up the ante, bleeding at times for what I saw as self-sacrifice, and still nothing from my parents. But here, I was somebody, and everyone liked what they saw.

We continued to grow the corporation, and the next step was to hire officers. An initial meeting was set up with new hire Peter Solomon in San Francisco. Fresh off a government-funded project not unlike my Synaptic Link Telehealth, he was dressed formally and very articulate. As I explained the company to him, he immediately recognized that Synaptic Link Telehealth was strong in areas where the government project had been lacking. We each saw the benefits of working with each other. He had graduated from an Ivy League university with honors and had been stationed in the Middle East as an army lieutenant. In addition, he was incredible with numbers and had too many business accomplishments to list. Initially, he had asked for a salary of $10,000.00 a month, which we couldn't accommodate yet. Fortunately, he agreed to work with us until we were able to secure more funding or make him a partner. We were extremely lucky to have Peter on board as a new asset, and I quickly got busy trying to raise more capital.

I started with our landlords, Christina and Brian Fang. Full-blown entrepreneurs, the Fangs had amassed over $100 million in assets. Despite this, they were kind, regular people who drove Teslas and Hondas. I invited them over for lunch that Saturday and made sure Vlad and Peter were in attendance. We decided to stick with just a soft pitch that day so they didn't think we had only invited them over to ask for money. We relied on Peter's eloquence to do most of the talking, as I tried to stay on top of Aileen and her kids to make sure they didn't cause any embarrassment.

After lunch, the Fangs told us they would get us in touch with some of their friends in the tech space locally. We were enthralled. We were on our way up and couldn't be more excited. To this day, I still wonder what the Fangs saw in us. Did they see strung-out, mentally ill drug addicts from New York riding on seed funding and a dream? Did they see an accomplished psychiatric nurse practitioner on his way to damnation?

The project moved along into December 2017, when our funding began to run low again. Software development ground to a halt. At this point, one of three things needed to happen: either we needed significant investment dollars, to secure a partnership, or to start launching the platform with a network of participating providers. With little time to make the decision, someone new entered the company, and things took a turn I could have never expected.

Jason Hendrix was an eight-time CEO with multiple successful company exits under his belt. His current role was as president of an insurance company headquartered in Manhattan. He didn't find me by accident; his business partner was a powerful attorney from back home in Upstate New York, with strong ties to local entrepreneurs. Turns out Jason had been watching us from afar all along and waiting for exactly the right time to step in (when we were just about out of money). With no other options on the table, he knew we didn't have much of a choice. He gave me a call in late December. The phone call lasted for almost 90 minutes as he grilled me on every part of the company, down to how the software itself worked. We ended the call with plans for a follow-up the next week. I couldn't believe such a successful CEO was interested in me or my company, and this inflated my ego even more. To boot, we did a tour of the software platform, after which he said, "This is better than 98% of what is on the market." I had engineered it just from my own mind, no external help.

In the meantime, we couldn't slow down. Somehow, Vlad had acquired two tickets to TechCrunch, an elite convention where investors go to view cutting-edge tech startup companies. With uncompleted software, we were up against companies that had been around for years. Nevertheless, we loaded our pitch decks and arrived at the convention in full business attire. A massive screen at the convention center displayed our company's listing with our names and titles. Over 10,000 people, including influential entrepreneurs, saw my name listed as a CEO! This was a massive dopamine hit and all I could think about was going further, gaining more recognition, and making it big in a way my parents would finally be forced to acknowledge.

Truthfully, we were a minnow among sharks at TechCrunch. Some of the most impressive tech companies I had ever seen were in attendance. Companies had flown in from all over the world to present, and some of them had been working on their software for up to fifteen years before unveiling it here. One of the crowning projects was presented by a team of Russians who had flown in. They had worked for over a decade on software that took your picture and then displayed what you would look like in each outfit while shopping online for clothes. Amazon previously had a similar product, but this company had spent years improving on it. They would no doubt blow up and get acquired after presenting here. Imagine working on something for a decade and then being set for life. In my mind, that was my entire reason for doing all of this (at least, that's what I told myself to justify my actions and behaviors).

While on the convention hall floor, we were able to pitch to interested entrepreneurs and investors. Despite my flawless pitch deck, we had yet to make any connections. People weren't looking to invest in something that wasn't making money yet. Nevertheless, we saw presenting at TechCrunch as a major accomplishment, something that would legitimize us in the business and tech worlds. We were still gaining momentum, I told myself. Once again, I was really just pursuing validation and dopamine hits. In the background of all this, I was abusing people, drugs, and my prescriptive privileges to continue the journey. Many of these new people who came into my life were looking to use me to obtain drugs, and I was looking to use them to obtain fame and fortune. I continued to leverage Adderall, cocaine, and money to further my work. In my mind, that was just how things worked in the world of business; I knew executives of major Fortune 500's that abused the shit out of Adderall and cocaine! The difference for me was that I had too much access and no moderation. Remember, I'm crazy, so the dopamine lift from Adderall and cocaine acted as an antidepressant for me (something I was not used to). It did for Freud too.

Two weeks later, Peter and I reconvened for a meeting with Jason. Peter had navigated many startup environments in the past, and he expressed his thoughts and desires for a partnership with Jason going forward. Jason could see the value Peter brought to the company, as he brought out flawless spreadsheets with 10-year projections. Nothing shy of a numbers genius, Peter demonstrated how changing one number on the first spreadsheet would cause a cascade of calculations and correctly populate numbers accordingly on every subsequent spreadsheet. By the end of the meeting, Synaptic Link Telehealth was partnered with Jason's Manhattan insurance company.

That month, January 2018, I flew back to New York to present the company to the Nurse Practitioners Association at a luxurious country club in Southfield, the town I used to live in with Abbie. I rented a nice house on Airbnb for the week and spent most of each day working on corporate matters, but without Aileen on my back I was able to enjoy the local nightlife.

Aileen and the kids stayed behind in California, so I spent my first night in New York with some old friends at the strip club she used to work at. I had a full script of Adderall and had just scored an eight ball of coke. I was pretty blitzed by midnight when we arrived at the club. Girls would come by our table when word got around that we were loaded with C&C, cash and cocaine. It was exactly what they were looking for. Eventually, a girl walked by who I immediately recognized as Aileen's rival from her days working here. The girl gave me a look in passing that I immediately understood. It was like a new drug had hit the table and I had to have her. The only trick would be getting out of here with her without club management noticing. If girls slept with club patrons, they ran the risk of getting fired.

At this point, you might be asking yourself how I could bring myself to cheat on Aileen, knowing that I would be flying home to rejoin life with her and her kids at the end of the week. Normally, I am not the cheating type; doing so weighs heavily on my conscience. But "cheating" on Aileen was not the same as cheating on Abbie. Aileen had been sleeping around on me with idiots from her hometown since two weeks into our relationship. She was unaware that I even knew, but she had left her phone unlocked one day as she took a shower. In fact, she never got off dating and hookup websites after we got into a relationship. After taking this into account, sleeping with her sworn enemy felt justified.

Lockwood

We met up at my Airbnb every night that week. It was amazing, but I could tell by the look on her face that the enjoyment for her was on another level. Aileen was a bully, and had made nights miserable for this girl when they worked together. She was getting off on the fact that Aileen was thousands of miles away, and there was nothing she could do about this. We were both using each other, she was using me for revenge and I was using her for sex, but we didn't care. The temporary arrangement worked out great.

That week, I worked alongside Jason and his subordinates as we prepared for meetings with the heads of hospitals, healthcare companies, clinics, etc. These were all small events leading up to the main event, the NPA meeting at the country club. While I presented, the plan was to have Jason and his entourage sitting in the back so they could get a read on how everyone was responding to the presentation. Since these were my own people I would be presenting to, other nurse practitioners, I wasn't worried about how they would react. I was correct: the event went off without a hitch, I killed the presentation, and I ended the night swarmed with my peers all clamoring to get on board with my project. I don't know if my colleagues believed in me or wanted to share the spotlight. Either way, they understood the presentation, even the ones who didn't like me and signed up that night to pilot the platform.

*　　　*　　　*

After the intense week of work and extracurriculars, I flew back to California. My first night back, Aileen cornered me to discuss something important. Exhausted and burnt-out, I was completely unreceptive to the idea of having a "talk". She insisted, and I found myself standing in front of her on our porch overlooking the beautiful view of San Francisco. Time stopped and everything went sideways as she broke the news to me that, for the second time, I was going to be a father. I was in disbelief. She claimed she was on birth control. Well, it turns out that she had stopped taking her birth control pills when we arrived in California and neglected to tell me. I was suddenly enraged at the thought of this whore having my child. This was absolutely not part of my plan; I didn't want another child and this would extinguish any future possibility of Abbie and I getting back together.

The devastating news caused my evil to reach far beyond the walls of our Portola Valley mansion. I suddenly found myself threatening Abbie back on the East Coast, insisting I was going to take Giovanni with me to California. I was completely off my rocker. Fortunately, she remained level-headed and knew to ignore my tantrums. Drugs and delusions of grandeur owned me. Looking back, I believe that Aileen's pregnancy caused me to push Abbie away. I didn't want her to get hurt further, and I knew the news would affect her. I was hurting, too, and the only thing I knew how to do was viciously go on the offensive.

No matter what I did or where I went, I was locked into an endless cycle of pain. Aileen's outbursts grew more violent and vicious towards me, and the relationship spiraled into a loop of domestic violence. This pushed me further into drug addiction. Russell Brand talked about how pain and addiction are linked using a five-point model of the cycle of addiction:

1. Pain
2. The usage of an addictive agent to lessen or distract from the pain (this could be anything: drugs, sex, food, work, codependency)
3. Temporary distraction from the source of pain
4. Consequences of using the addictive agent
5. Guilt leads to low self-esteem and more pain

Basically, addiction begins with pain and leads to more pain, ultimately perpetuating the cycle. When you give in to the initial pain, you lose your focus, which directly leads to the irrational and illogical decision to abuse drugs. Abuse or addiction becomes a repetitive behavior that occurs despite the obvious mental and physical consequences. As for me, I failed right at step one. Since I hadn't yet identified my source of pain, I ended up both addicted to drugs and behaving in ways that a sane individual would never do. One of these behaviors was my relationship with Aileen. I was in pain when I first met Aileen, who provided sex and drugs which allowed me a distraction only to repeat those behaviors, and feeling more and more guilty every time. The guilt was that I abandoned Abbie and

Giovanni and fatherhood. That guilt was scathing pain that caused the cycle to repeat.

Being codependent is strange in that it allows for a certain acceptable level of pain as long as the other person is in your life. It's kind of like being addicted to drugs, and the consequences of a codependent relationship can be just as bad. Both Aileen and I were codependent, which is a bad combination. This led to the violence reinforcing the relationship: a big, violent blow-up would happen and one of us would decide to "end the relationship". This would immediately lead to the other falling in line and doing whatever it took to make up, despite how bad the initial atrocity committed was. We were both addicted to drugs as well as addicted to the relationship, so our foundation was anything but stable. But we were both codependent, so we thrived off the idea of having someone there all the time. As a future CPS worker would put it, we were "toxic at best".

There was nothing special about Aileen in particular, but I subconsciously knew that my relationship with her and her three children was my way of showing the world that I was capable of having a "normal" family. I even told a marriage counselor that they were my "rental family" ...almost like I was just practicing on them, and once I had "achieved" perfect fatherhood I would return to Abbie and Giovanni and we would flourish. I sought validation as a provider, husband, and father from someone who only thrived in chaos. Of course it was never going to happen, but I couldn't see it at the time. I just kept trying to get it "right."

Aileen had a lot of issues of her own. She spoke of being raped at a young age before going into the foster system and eventually getting adopted by a well-off family of intellectuals. Despite this, she ended up with only her GED. She has stories of being in school and pretending to be much dumber than she was so they wouldn't expect her to think or complete assignments. The only form of validation she wanted was physical, so she never had any real career aspirations (although she presented as marginalized white population that needed to be rescued and was very easily impressed by the most basic displays of wealth, I later found out that her wealthy adoptive father would hand her wads of cash any time she asked and pay any bills she needed. She was never really "poor").

As a teenager and young adult, she was very promiscuous. She became a stripper by choice, not out of necessity. Her life revolved around validation from men, and she gave them her attention very freely, even when in a committed relationship (she had a way of playing dumb and apologizing that always seemed to get her off the hook). Despite this, she hated men. In the strip club, she saw herself as predator, not prey. One time, she told me that the attention she got as a stripper was just as good as the money, and the attention was even better if the guy was married. I didn't make the connection at the time, but I think that was what originally drew her into a relationship with me. Looking back, in the early days of our relationship, she would do anything she could to get in the way of any communication I had with Abbie.

*   *   *

Meanwhile, things continued with the corporation. The partnership with Jason's insurance company became official, and, on February 2, 2018, we moved back to New York. Upon arriving back in New York, we moved into a beautiful townhouse. I received 1 million preferred stock in the new company that had been formed as a result of the partnership. This meant that upon acquisition I could become an overnight millionaire. Lord knows I had earned it. I already sacked a marriage and son for the cause. Aileen, excited at the prospect of a wealthy life, was just about in her second trimester now. I reopened my psych practice with a colleague, in a building kitty-corner to the new headquarters for Synaptic Link Telehealth. I quickly re-established supply lines for Adderall so I could work the 18-hour days that felt necessary at the time. Aileen perceived all the time I spent at work as abandonment, and she would punish me severely whenever I was at home. Unbeknownst to me, she had even taken it upon herself to contact some of my patients to let them know how "unacceptable" it was that I was talking to them for so long. Any and all attention had to be on her at all times. Anything else was abandonment in her mind.

As the days passed, I felt more and more guilty for bringing a child into the world with her after I had abandoned Giovanni. For a while, I kept my appointments to visit with him on Sundays, whether my head was swimming with cocaine and Adderall or not. Sometimes I had gone days without sleep before visiting him and could barely keep it together. On one visit, we were swimming indoors while Abbie supervised from the benches. I came up from being underwater and two white streams began pouring from my nose. Thank God she was so unfamiliar with drugs that she had no idea what was going on. That should have been a wake-up call for me, but I ignored it, continuing to use drugs and work tirelessly at my practice and the corporation. I continued the cycle like *clockwork* of a certain color.

As Aileen's due date drew near, I became more and more despondent. My visits with Giovanni became less and less frequent before ceasing entirely. Finally, on the day she went into labor, I tried to kill myself again. She was out of the house and her ex-husband's parents were watching the three children at their house. I sat in a dark room and put on sad music, consuming narcotics and alcohol. I couldn't believe I was bringing a child into this world with such an evil creature. This wasn't my plan. All I could think about was my ex-wife and how I had abandoned Giovanni. I didn't want to live, I didn't want a child with Aileen. My relationship with her was only supposed to be temporary.

By the time Aileen found me, I was deeply sedated. She somehow got me into the car and drove us to the hospital. By this point, she was in active labor. I don't remember much after she got admitted to the hospital. I was on the brink of respiratory depression when Dr. Cohen, who happened to be the on-call OB, came into the room where I was sitting. He knew I had been struggling with this for some time and wanted to be there for me. After this, I remember wandering the L&D unit before leaving the hospital. I crossed the street and purchased half a dozen Boston Cream donuts for no apparent reason.

I woke up shortly after on the hospital lawn, with the donuts pressed to my shirt. In a daze, I entered the hospital, past security, and ended up in the room where Aileen was being monitored. Intense labor had begun, and the room was filled with nurses, the anesthesia team, and the OB. Abbie's friend from graduate school was at the helm with anesthesia and said hello to me, an uncomfortable memory that my brain somehow logged with perfect clarity. Everyone was encouraging Aileen to push as I stood nearby, dissociated, completely out of it, as I watched my second son come into the world. Scissors were thrust into my hands to cut the umbilical cord, which I somehow managed, despite seeing triple at that point.

After this, I became agitated and belligerent as I realized this was the same hospital where Giovanni was born. I told the nurses I didn't want my name on the birth certificate. After seeing Aileen's negative reaction to this, I decided I had better man up and take responsibility for my creation. After all, it wasn't my son that I resented, it was the fact that it was with her. *What have I done? What have I done?* cycled on repeat through my brain. This was one of the first real, tangible consequences of my actions, and it definitely wouldn't be the last. I had the distinct feeling that I had peaked in my journey, and it would all be downhill from here.

Aileen's three children were brought into her room to hold their new baby brother. Aileen had no problem breastfeeding and was able to leave the hospital in a day or two. I arrived back home to find I was unsurprisingly behind on work with both my practice and the corporation. Trying to be nice, Jason texted me a baby emoji. I simply replied, "It's a boy." I didn't feel like the world was happy for me. It felt like everyone knew that this baby was nothing more than a point of leverage for Aileen to control me, haunt me, get money out of me, etc., as part of her devious plan. As she would tell a friend of mine a few years later while giggling, "I kind of tricked him into having a baby with me so he would be tied to me!" She actually thought this was a funny, cute story to be shared amongst friends.

No congratulatory messages came from my family. They purposely went away to Maine the week of Aileen's due date and took Abbie and Giovanni with them. If that doesn't spell out that what I had done was unacceptable, I don't know what does. In fact, they wouldn't even meet baby Lorenzo for a couple of years. It was around this time that people in my professional and social lives began to pull back from me as well. It seemed like everyone knew that Aileen was dangerous, and now that she was postpartum and stressed, the chances of a centennial event increased.

Diapers, Delusions, and a Damn Good Setup

Aileen experienced her first episode of postpartum psychosis about two and a half weeks after Lorenzo was born. It was a Thursday, and I was finishing up at Synaptic Link Telehealth headquarters at about 10:00 p.m.. Since we were sharing one car at the time, Aileen came to pick me up. The car ride home was uneventful, and I was looking forward to having dinner at home and hopefully getting some sleep. I had no idea that Aileen had resumed abusing Adderall after giving birth and hadn't slept at all.

We got home, and, just like every other night, we filled our water bottles and grabbed something small from the fridge before settling into the master bedroom. I noticed that Lorenzo was becoming colicky and fussing quite a bit. At that point, I had been up for three days, and it was definitely beginning to affect me negatively. I tried to think of the responsible thing to do. "Hey, I think I'm going to sleep downstairs on the couch tonight. Lorenzo's crying a lot and I really need to get some sleep tonight, I've been up with you for days."

Calmly but firmly, Aileen replied, "You don't want to sleep with me?" Suddenly, I saw her eyes shift shades of green and silver with a glare I had never seen before. My gut instinct immediately led me to think this was some form of psychosis, but in all my years of work I had never come across postpartum mood issues in this way. Aileen held Lorenzo in her arms, and my eyes immediately shot to his head flopping up and down as she wasn't supporting it. She began ranting, and I could tell she wasn't even registering the danger that he was in. I immediately jumped into save and protect mode, catching her by surprise to swiftly but carefully grab him from her clutches.

This triggered her further, and she started yelling about how I was abusing her and hurting Lorenzo. Unbeknownst to me, Aileen's oldest kid heard the commotion from downstairs and used Siri to call 911. The kids were used to Aileen and her ex-husband getting into violent fights and thought that this was more of the same. Aileen continued to rant and scream while I tried in vain to de-escalate the situation. I was standing in my bedroom in my underwear holding my son, and suddenly I heard my full name being shouted from downstairs. "ASHER

LOCKWOOD, COME DOWN WITH YOUR HANDS UP." Aileen suddenly had a devious look in her eye and a wicked grin to match. I sighed, handing her Lorenzo before walking downstairs with my hands up, still in my underwear.

The town cops brought me outside and beat my ass in the parking lot before ordering me to get dressed. I was cuffed and brought to the local police station for booking. I tried to explain to everyone I came across that Aileen was experiencing serious postpartum psychosis, and was alone with a baby. No one took me seriously. One of the officers had gone through the house and found the makeshift room Aileen had set up without my knowledge in the basement furnace room; she had strewn about cut-up photos of Abbie and Giovanni. Still, no one seemed concerned, even though postpartum psychosis was and is a serious medical emergency.

I ended up cuffed to a desk for hours without food, water, or anyone talking to me. The officer who finally decided to process me hit me with five felony counts and a restraining order. By the time he finished booking me, it was 2:00 a.m., and I needed to be detained until I was to be arraigned in the morning by a DA. This meant I was to be taken to the county correctional facility, where they stripped me down, took my prints and pictures, and put me in an orange jumpsuit. Was this for real? Soon, I was in a cell with what had to have been the biggest guy I had ever seen, but he was cool and left me alone. Someone brought me a tray with food, which I refused. I was so exhausted from the whole ordeal, as well as the previous days without sleep, that I was able to pass out until they got me the next morning to prepare for the hearing with the DA.

I was quickly introduced to my public defender, a fat, stuttering man, before being brought before the Judge. She looked at me, evaluated the situation for herself, and showed mercy, letting me "go on my own recognizance." I was soon released, and it immediately hit me that I had no car or home due to the restraining order. I used my phone to call an Uber to take me to a hotel on the other side of town. I was trying to avoid, not just Aileen, but Jason. As an executive officer in a company, I knew my title and stake in the corporation were at risk if word were to get out that I was involved in any kind of criminal activity. Not only that, but my APRN license could be at risk depending on how this all shook out.

Lockwood

I couldn't believe Aileen would do this to me, she knew that criminal charges would put our livelihood in jeopardy. Was she really this vindictive? She had given a statement saying I was far from coherent, which she thought would hurt me, but actually wound up helping me in the long run. It was at this point that I knew that I was on my own and that I needed to establish myself in a new residence, away from her. I decided to stay in a hotel for the time being, and I reached out to some friends I knew who were criminal defense attorneys because I needed to ensure these five felony charges wouldn't stick. Too much was riding on me.

Time away from Aileen was good for me; both old friends and girls came out of the woodwork to hang out when they heard the news that I was away from her. I wouldn't find out until later, but Aileen was doing some socializing of her own, namely, sleeping with her ex-husband as well as trying to find rich, connected men to establish herself with. One such local politician she was fucking bought $5,000.00 worth of Christmas presents for her kids that year.

Meanwhile, Jason had sent minions out to try and find me since I had gone dark as far as the corporation was concerned. They had gotten as close as actually staying in the same hotel as me, but we never crossed paths. Luckily for me, Jason had to purchase my intellectual property, as per our Dentons lawyers, to the tune of my credit card debt. The money came just in time. While I did use some to settle up some credit cards, I also put several months down on a new luxury condo. The place was beautiful: tall wooden doors, granite countertops, two huge bathrooms, and my own garage. Best of all, it was only five minutes from my office and Synaptic Link Telehealth headquarters. My financial mistake was paying some of the credit card tabs in full. They'll settle for pennies on the dollar so don't give them shit.

It felt like I was entering a new chapter of my life, and I decided to just focus on myself. For the first time, I could have my own thoughts, completely uninterrupted or impeded. It was extremely foreign to me, but I liked it. It wouldn't be long until I began searching for the next dopamine spike in the form of a girl, however.

*   *   *

Adderall and Other False Prophets

With Aileen no longer a part of my day-to-day life and a nice place all to myself, I had a void to fill in my life. Instead of using this time to look inward and work on myself, I wound up focusing on another addictive entity: spending drug-sprinkled nights at the local strip clubs. I know, I know...I did this before and look where it got me. My father always used to say, "Asher, you always have to learn the hard way," which usually led to me getting spanked. I was determined to live my "single life" to the fullest, and sure as hell I did (to the tune of $100,000.00 in cocaine purchases that year).

I was living about ten minutes from a strip club called the Velvet Room (VR) and five minutes from work. I would see patients during the day, and at night I would go to VR all alone and spend about $500.00-$1,000.00 on the girls. I was surviving on Adderall and protein shakes and nothing else. I hadn't been able to find cocaine for some time until I bumped into a guy with the street name Buddah. It really felt like the universe at work the day I first met him in the bathroom at VR, a place one doesn't really meet strangers.

Buddah knew exactly what I wanted and could tell I had the cash to back it up. He told me to meet him in the back row of the parking lot in ten minutes. At the agreed-upon time, I stepped out to have a cigarette and saw three identical blacked-out SUVs backed into spots as far away from the building as possible. I approached the one in the center and could see two huge dudes in the front seats. The doors unlocked, and I hopped up into the backseat to see Buddah sitting there. He gave me a big hello and produced a bag of cocaine, as promised.

$350.00 later, I was high as a kite and loving life. Technically, I overpaid for the shit, but I wanted guaranteed snow and not some stomped-on crap. I could tell that this stuff was good (isn't the first bag always the best?). With the newfound fourfold increase in dopamine in my cortex, I was king of the evening. Combined with the Adderall I already had on board, I was feeling great and couldn't be stopped.

Buddah and I grew closer. He would sometimes stop by my office for drops, as by that point, I was running exclusively on drugs. Eventually, we started to hang out outside of cocaine deals. VR continued to be a favorite hangout spot; I ended up sleeping with quite a few of the strippers there (some I paid, some were just for fun or for sport). We would also meet up at my place or at his big house on 87th Ave in the shady part of town. We grew so close that one day, he shared something personal with me.

He sat me down for a conversation and explained to me that he was a Crip, and the big house he lived in was one of many on that street outfitted with top security and exit strategies. He showed me the huge garbage can they kept filled with bleach. In the event of a raid, they could throw an entire kilo in there and it would dissolve instantly. The street was one of the major veins in the local Crip organization, with each house on the street producing $50k a week in crack-cocaine sales. Yeh, it was kind of serious.

I became such a fixture on 87th Ave that Buddah ended up getting me my own parking space, as well as affixing a blue flag inconspicuously to the back left part of my car. It was just like Snoop Dogg said: *"I keep a blue flag hangin' out my backside. But only on the left side, yeah, that's the Crip side."* I felt like one of the guys. They were very easy to hang out with, and to my surprise, very smart and knowledgeable. We had deep conversations about everything from religion to politics to the economy to stories of incarceration.

I estimate that I did about $100,000.00 in cocaine that year. I had nothing but money and time on my hands, and no Aileen. Well, I say that with a wink and a nudge. Aileen and I were actually speaking again and she would frequently drop by my place late at night when I was done with the clubs and partying. She would bring little Lorenzo, and I later found out she was leaving her other three young kids home alone. We'd party together into the wee hours of the morning, sometimes going through the entire next day.

One of my favorite things to do after these long evenings was to hang a bag of IV fluid with shots of Toradol. After one of those bags you felt like a million bucks, absolutely amazing. The only problem was that my hands were usually shaking due to drug use and lack of sleep. I usually always managed to get the catheter in the vein, but sometimes I would miss and spend hours trying to hit the vessel. This always took place during the hours of 6:00-11:00 a.m., yet another thing to focus on that wasn't myself. When there's not a single moment where you're thinking rationally or logically, it's easy to miss exactly how neck-deep you are in insanity. The frog and boiling water scenario.

Buddah and I were so close that he even held baby Lorenzo at a party I was throwing at my place. It was at this party where he first met Aileen, even though she was wasted at the time. After they met, he leaned in close to me and said "You know who the most dangerous gangster in the room is...Aileen." How he had come to that conclusion only two minutes after meeting her is beyond me. I brushed off the warning, although time would prove him to be 100% correct.

Buddah wasn't the only gang member I was hanging out with during this chapter of my life. Ashley, one of the dancers at VR, had been with a Latin King for years. Ramon had grown up in Compton and committed his first homicide at age 16. This guy was no joke. He had spent years in solitary and used the time to read every religious text available. He was incredibly intelligent, and just as dangerous, if not more so, as Buddah and his counterparts. He would pimp his girl out to johns and would shoot her up with dope beforehand so the memory would be dulled. I ended up spending some time at Ramon's apartment with my friend Nathan, who was my IT guy at the time. Nathan was dangerous in his own way, especially with computers. He was a master of the dark net and was capable of things like wholesale purchase orders of illicit schedule one substances or emptying entire financial accounts into untraceable crypto accounts.

Despite the deadly cast of characters I was surrounding myself with, Aileen was still the most dangerous one in the room. Even Ramon took the time to come to my apartment one day and sit me down, saying that she wanted to see me "hanging and squirming". This was yet another warning I failed to heed; I was still blind to what she was doing and how she was doing it. I didn't believe him and continued my relationship with her. I mean, we had a kid together, of course I was going to stay! On top of that I owned Lorenzo on paper, having traded $25,000.00 for a stiff full custody that she agreed to in family court. Yes she sold him to me.

This is a good time to reflect on this point in my life. As you can see, without a solid reference point in life and knowing who you really are, the self becomes sculpted by the surrounding environment and the individuals one is surrounded with. In this state, choices you make are not really your own, even though you may perceive them to be. Without a solid set of personal principles setting parameters on your decisions, the outcomes of those decisions become chaotic, unpredictable, and harmful. Even Ramon had figured this out, since he had a lot of time to work on himself and reflect on his life's decisions. In the end, he may have chosen to continue to be a gangster, but at least he knew *why*. He also knew enough about human nature to see Aileen for what she really was, and to warn me, even though he didn't have to. In reality, the storm of chaos and destruction she caused was only just beginning.

*   *   *

Around this time, I was practicing out of an office about 5 minutes away from where I lived. The other provider I shared the office with was a good friend of mine who was an LMHC (and a very good one at that). She was very astute, but anyone could have seen that I was circling the drain. The amount of weight I had dropped was so drastic and unhealthy that people were no longer politely ignoring it and I started getting concerned comments. I didn't show up to the vast majority of my patients' appointments, and my colleague had to cover for me more and more. She became so concerned that she called the local police department for a wellness check on me. I was pissed at having to deal with the cops yet again. She suggested that maybe it was my dad who made the call. I didn't know any better at the time, so I bought it. I was also preoccupied with Aileen and the kids suddenly moving back in with me (more on that in a minute).

While I was in my drug- and insanity-filled bubble, the rest of the world was getting hit hard by COVID. My colleague and I decided to call it a day on our joint practice and broke ties as per her wish. I really couldn't blame her. I packed up my things and went home to begin setting up a home office so I could work solo taking telehealth patients. At first, working from home was great. Very quickly, however, it turned into another avenue for Aileen to try and exert control over me. I no longer had an office to escape to, we were stuck at home with each other 24/7. She interfered with my sessions with patients because she didn't like that my attention was on someone who wasn't her. The kids were also home all the time because the schools were shut down. Without the built-in structure and routine that school provided, the kids were acting like kids and there wasn't enough space in the apartment for me to find a quiet space away from everything for work. I couldn't focus and I moved my home office setup into the garage.

A few months earlier, while we were living apart, CPS had opened a case on Aileen for leaving her three young children home alone. What she neglected to share with me was that I was, by extension, included in the investigation. She also intentionally provided CPS with an incorrect address for me, so I never got the paperwork. In March of 2020, her restraining order against me expired, so she moved back in along with all four kids into my beautiful two-bedroom apartment.

Nathan had been living in my garage for a little bit, so things were already tighter than normal when she and the kids moved in. Nathan's presence in my house quickly became a grinding point for me and Aileen. She didn't like all the time I spent in the garage with him working on computer stuff for my practice because that was time that I wasn't giving her attention. She wanted him gone and was constantly on my ass about it.

After constant nagging, she decided to take action to force Nathan out of the house. It was early morning on Thursday or Friday, and Nathan and I had been awake all week working. It was finally time to pass out, and I was so exhausted that I actually found myself laying on the floor as I felt sleep slip over me like a heavy blanket. Immediately, I was violently shaken awake by Aileen. She actually continued to shake me as she started barking orders; she insisted that she had caught Nathan trying to look at her while she was changing and I needed to do something about it NOW.

I stood up, exhausted and disoriented, trying to parse what she was saying. Her tone became more demanding and I felt my level of agitation rising. Since I was so sleep deprived and had been jolted awake by her shaking me, I was running entirely on adrenaline with zero rational thought taking place. I hadn't even processed the actual accusation she was making yet. All I wanted was for her to stop talking and leave me the fuck alone. I was basically on autopilot at that point, willing to do whatever it would take to make her stop. I felt something taking control over me, almost as if I was possessed.

Lockwood

Aileen was still going on and on as I walked through the house in a trance to get to the garage to take care of business. I was basically incapable of thought at this point, although rage was building within me more and more with each word out of her mouth. Aileen was glued to my side, still goading me even as I stood in the garage. Her words were poison, hijacking my vulnerable mind like a virus. It didn't strike me as off until later, how, she didn't seem like someone who had just experienced something violating; she didn't even seem upset at all. Instead, she was gleeful with anticipation for the impending beatdown. She was enthralled at the chaotic situation she had orchestrated and the control she was exerting.

Long story short, Nathan ended up in a cast at the hospital. Fortunately, Nathan had known me for long enough at that point to know who I was, who I wasn't, and (maybe most importantly) who Aileen was. He declined to press charges. Per usual, Aileen had gotten exactly what she wanted, the removal of Nathan from my garage. Now she could abuse me without witnesses.

I didn't think things could possibly get more chaotic at that point but of course they did. About a month after Aileen and the kids moved in, CPS swarmed my apartment with police officers. They threw me out of the building and ordered me to go to rehab. I was completely flanked. I ended up heading to a motel in an Uber to wait for my departure to rehab. Apparently, Aileen had decided to get back at me for going to the strip club by using the family court system; unbeknownst to me, she had been submitting false claims about me to CPS for months.

The rehab I was heading to was in Pennsylvania, for anonymity. The driver for my trip was a retired colonel. The first half of our drive down was filled with engaging conversation as he regaled me with stories of his time in the army and told me all about how he came into the job of picking up addicts to bring to 30-day inpatient rehab. He put me at ease, and I began to relax and enjoy the ride until my phone suddenly lit up.

It was a text from Aileen notifying me that, not only was she still seeing her ex-husband, but that he was going to be around for the entire month I was to be gone. I immediately began to freak out and knew I had to get back to New York immediately if I was going to be able to head this off. If I had been in my right mind at the time, I would have realized that her bullshit was nothing compared to the wrath I could potentially face from the court and my state boards if I didn't complete this rehab stay. Not to mention the fact that I was currently fully addicted to both Adderall and cocaine, which was enough of a reason to dry out. Neither of these thoughts occurred to me, and I entered the facility with the complete wrong mindset.

I arrived at the facility in the evening. They searched me and immediately put me into detox, even though I was stable. For some reason, they decided to withhold all of my psychiatric medications. This sent me into withdrawal and gave me one of the worst headaches of my life, which they decided to treat with ibuprofen and not the psych meds I needed. After being in the facility for three days, I was sent to meetings where the topic of conversation and counsel was entirely based on the needs of alcoholics and contained nothing that applied to me. I finally decided that this place wasn't a good fit for me and told the nurses I wanted to leave AMA (against medical advice).

I couldn't sleep that night and asked the nursing staff for a clipboard and loose paper. I sat there and began writing the story of my current situation. Words flowed out of my hand and I spent hours getting it all out; how, once upon a time, I was happily married, how it all fell apart, how I met the wrong person, and everything Aileen had done to further my suffering and land me in my current predicament. The nursing staff read it, all 36 pages, and thought it was a great story with a lot of personal insight into my situation. The next day, the therapist assigned to me took it and used it as evidence that I was not stable and in need of further rehabilitation. Was she right? Looking back, she was. However, how she went about it was extremely unprofessional – calling me profanities in front of other patients and so on.

Despite this, I met with the administration to try and secure my exit. The woman I spoke with was initially kind and understanding, but became irritable and nasty upon reading the reports from CPS. I pushed the issue, and she became more irate by the minute until I finally asked security to call me a cab back to New York. They couldn't deny this as I had technically entered the facility voluntarily. I could tell the woman was livid that I was able to afford the $650.00 cab fare back home and she chided me throughout the entire process of getting myself signed out.

Lockwood

My cab driver was extremely talkative and we smoked throughout the first part of the ride. Sometime about halfway through the drive, I must have fallen asleep. I woke up in my driveway and entered my condo, which was dark and empty. Aileen soon showed up with baby Lorenzo, even though she wasn't supposed to be near me as per CPS (while I was in rehab, CPS put her in a women's shelter with Lorenzo). Per usual, she did not recognize authority and did what she wanted to do despite the consequences (which, at that time, would have been removal of Lorenzo). This continued for a month or two, sneaking around to see each other in secret despite what CPS commanded.

Even though they had sent police to my apartment and demanded I go to rehab, I still wasn't taking my involvement in the CPS case seriously. I still had yet to receive any paperwork from them addressed to me (refer back to my previous statement about Aileen providing them with an incorrect address for me; since the initial case was opened back when her and I weren't living together, I assume that she possibly thought she could hide it from me for a while by giving them false info for me), and when they tried to talk to me, I would stonewall them. I had plenty of other things going on and I mostly wanted to be left alone so I could do drugs in peace. This would eventually turn into 6 years of endless investigations, court dates, random drug tests and months-long domestic violence, anger, and parenting classes. Funny enough, as soon as I finally left her in 2023, all the requirements and mandates from family court pertaining to me vanished. While I was in the middle of this storm of chaos, paranoid from drug use and lack of sleep, I always truly believed that we were being unfairly (and possibly illegally) harassed and targeted by CPS. Now, I can look back and truly understand why CPS was pressing so hard: Aileen is an abusive and neglectful mother.

After a month or so, Aileen and Lorenzo were allowed to move back in with me (her other three kids were placed in the care of her ex-husband's parents by CPS). Almost immediately, she started orchestrating events that led to the police being called. There were so many calls that the property manager let me know that they would not be renewing my lease. One time, she felt that I was spending too much time with Nathan in the garage (back when he lived with me), so she drove my car into the garage door. Other times, she literally tried to kill me.

Adderall and Other False Prophets

On one of those nights, we had just returned home after spending the evening together at the VR. Nothing had seemed out of the ordinary to me while we were at the club or on the drive home. My back was to her as we entered the house and passed into the kitchen. Out of nowhere, the hairs on the back of my neck stood up and I became filled with a strange dread. I turned around and my eyes immediately went to the large saucepan in her hands. Within a fraction of a second, she took a massive swing at my neck with the saucepan. I leaned back, *Matrix*-style, and the pan missed my neck by centimeters.

I immediately shifted into defense mode, with no time to try and figure out what had set her off. With the pan on the floor, she grabbed the closest potentially dangerous object: a massive cast iron pot. She launched the pot right at my head, and I ended up taking the hit to my forearm. Then she came at me with a large glass framed picture. I was fighting for my life; she was unpredictable and extremely dangerous.

I was somehow able to lock myself into a room without her, and I quickly called an attorney I was friends with. He called the police on my behalf to come do a check. When they arrived, she immediately slipped on her sociopath's mask to appear cool, calm and collected. The cops bought it and left. By that point, I was so exhausted that all I wanted to do was pass out. The next day, she acted like nothing had happened the night before. That was usually how things played out after things got violent. If you're reading this and wondering why I would stay with someone who tried to murder me, the answer is pain and drugs. When your judgment is clouded, you'll put up with things that are completely outside the realm of acceptable. When you're enough of a drug addict, anything goes, and I mean that.

Man Hunt in the Adirondacks

Nathan and I hadn't spoken since the garage incident, which meant that I was in desperate need of a new IT guy for my practice. I needed someone I could trust, so I turned to my circle for personal recommendations. The problem was that my circle consisted entirely of people you would not introduce to your grandmother. Nevertheless, I put out some feelers and one of the dancers at the VR actually knew someone who ran a local IT company she could put me in touch with. I agreed and set up a meeting with him at my place.

His name was Jose, and as soon as I met him, I could tell that he was a very smart and cunning individual. I explained what I was looking for help with (basically I wanted to automate certain parts of my solo practice in order to streamline and simplify the headache of all the necessary paperwork required for running a psych practice). He said he could definitely do that, and the conversation shifted to his fees. He laid out a pay scale that seemed very steep to me (upwards of $6000.00). He convinced me that the cost was commensurate with his experience and skills. He seemed invested in helping execute the vision I had for the practice, and I made my usual mistake of trusting up front.

Jose started working on the project we discussed, as well as his other ideas for how to make my practice run as smoothly as possible. Before long, I had even hired his ex-wife to work as my receptionist (she wasn't great at it, but at this point in time I was running through mediocre receptionists every few months because of how chaotic my life was). Jose soon came to me with a new setup for payment processing. My patient's payments would go into a PayPal account that he set up and had direct access to. I wasn't tracking the money going into that account, just the sums getting deposited into my checking account. As long as enough money kept flowing in to keep up with my habits, I was happy. Jose knew this and ended up taking advantage of it.

Things didn't work out with Jose's ex-wife as my receptionist, so I hired Alyssa as a replacement. Another VR special, she was a stripper with three kids. Like me, she also happened to be an amphetamine addict. It helped numb the pain she felt after suffering a stillbirth at eight months gestation as well as the divorce she was in the middle of. Despite all of this, she excelled at the job. I introduced Alyssa and Jose, and he was friendly enough to her at first. I think he was trying to sniff around to see if she knew anything about his misdeeds.

Her first week on the job, she took a full inventory of my entire practice and discovered that Jose had been stealing thousands of dollars from me using the weird system he put in place. He assumed that, since I was so deep down the hole of drug addiction, that I would never find out or care that he was skimming so much from my accounts (in addition to the astronomical amounts he was charging me for the privilege of being robbed!). After Alyssa presented me with detailed breakdowns of everything Jose had embezzled, I decided to pay a visit to the office he worked in downtown.

Lo and behold, Jose's office was empty and he was nowhere to be found. The landlord happened to be on the property the day I visited, and I asked if he knew what happened or where Jose went. The only information he had was that the space Jose was leasing from him was recently vacated. He didn't have any leads on where I could find him. I eventually ended up being able to track him down with the help of an old friend, but I'll come back to that later.

Meanwhile, Alyssa continued to be a great addition to the practice and was able to juggle everything required for the role while taking care of her kids at the same time. She made it look easy, and I was impressed. We grew closer as time went on and she introduced me to her children. A few months of her working for me had gone by when she suddenly called me late one night. Something was wrong, one of her children had fallen and got injured. She knew I was a nurse, and she trusted me, so she asked if I could possibly come over and take a look at her child's injury to see if it needed medical attention or not. I told her I would be right over.

I could tell that something was off as soon as I stepped inside her house. The children were nowhere to be found and Alyssa was standing in front of a large fish tank. She was acting strange, kind of slowly dancing by herself while looking at the cell phone in her hand. Before I could confront her about where the supposedly injured child was, she pulled me into one of the bedrooms and tried to start seducing me. I got into the bed, still fully dressed, and I asked her about her husband and the divorce. She assured me that he was staying with family during the process.

Suddenly, I heard the front door open and a very angry-sounding male voice called out "Alyssa, where are you?!" I immediately started panicking. Without thinking, I leapt from the bed and crawled underneath it, trying to keep myself as tucked away and hidden as possible. I had never met her husband before and had no idea what to expect, but judging by his voice, he sounded large and very angry.

Alyssa got out of bed and went to greet him, but he wasn't interested. He saw my car in the driveway and just kept yelling "Where is he?! Where is he?!" Keeping as still as possible, I watched from under the bed as he paced around the room and down the hallway. I scanned the room for any possible exits and everything was a dead end. He knew he had me trapped in the house. Eventually, he came back into the bedroom to continue looking for me. He walked around the length of the bed and finally discovered where I was hiding, all 140 lbs. of me at that point. He told me to get up and I did, and I finally got a good look at him. He was about 6'2" and definitely had at least 100 lbs. on me. To my surprise, he didn't seem to want to fight. He just kept asking me if I was married. I answered truthfully, telling him that I was not married. Upon hearing that, he escorted me to the door, telling me to never come back here again, or else. Incredibly relieved to have avoided a fight, I got into my car and peeled out of her driveway. I ended up letting Alyssa go, with a nice bonus to help smooth things over. I never heard from either of them again, thankfully. I believe they were trying to set me up for something, but never fully understood what the end goal was.

Anyway, despite all the craziness that surrounded her leaving her job at the practice, she had still been the one to uncover Jose's embezzlement scheme. I think he had suspicions that Alyssa caught him and that his house of cards was about to fall, and that's why he abandoned his former office space and vanished without a trace. He wasn't responding to any phone calls or emails, and I was starting to get more and more pissed off at the situation. I needed to find him but kept running into dead ends. At this point, I realized I needed to bring in the big guns and I knew just the guy who would be able to track him down.

I knew this would be exactly the type of situation for Nathan to handle. He was incredibly skilled with tracking down people and information online. He could find literally anyone, and he enjoyed doing it. I laid out the situation to him in an email to see if he was on board, and he was. The hatchet had been buried and he forgave me, as evidenced by how eager he was to help me try and find Jose after I explained how he fucked me over.

Nathan quickly got to work on his laptop, using his skills that earned him the title King of the Internet. He was successful and was somehow able to locate Jose at a property approximately 90 minutes away, completely off the grid, in the middle of the Adirondack Mountains. Nathan and I immediately began forming a plan for payback. Needless to say, we were both doing drugs and not sleeping, and these factors heavily influenced the plan. At the time, however, it seemed flawless.

Finally, we had amassed all of our supplies and it was the big night. Nathan and I were fully suited up in camo and were strapped with spike strips and smoke grenades. We drove up through the mountains and parked my car in a densely wooded area that was far enough from the house so that he couldn't see or hear it, but close enough that we could run back there in a reasonably short time if we had to abort. From there, we walked the rest of the way.

Nathan had done plenty of recon, and we planned the best path to take from the car so that we would approach the house from the woods, never crossing the front of the house or stepping foot on the driveway or yard. We were stealthy, hiding in the big snowbanks that were made when the driveway was plowed. It was dark out, and Jose was a weird paranoid tech guy so I assumed his place would be loaded with cameras and other security equipment. We needed to be extremely slow and careful about this.

We hid motionless behind the snowbanks for what felt like forever. Finally, it was time to make a calculated, careful move. Nathan took the first step. As soon as his boot hit the ground, I began to make out an odd shape in the tree above us. Suddenly, the tree illuminated with a light so bright I was blinded for a few seconds. Nathan's movement had triggered a massive motion-activated floodlight that was mounted in the tree.

With the property now fully lit up, I could see exactly just how protected it was. Multiple cameras were mounted at every possible angle. Every tree had a floodlight in it, motion detectors were everywhere. Thousands of tiny red LEDs lit up across every possible surface as the movement triggered the cameras to activate.

My eyes flew to a silhouette in the window. It looked like Jose, but it was hard to make out exactly what he was carrying.

I flashed back to a conversation I had with Jose before he vanished. He explained how he was a huge gun collector and even pulled up some pictures on his phone of his very serious collection. We needed to get out of there, *immediately*. Nathan was still frozen in place after triggering the light. I barely poked my head around the snowbank, just enough to get his attention. He slowly turned his head towards me, unsure if any further movement would trigger an alarm or something worse. After a second of frantic eye contact, I mouthed *Run*.

We abandoned the mission and both took off into a full sprint. We didn't look back or slow down the entire mile back to where the car was hidden. We were both completely out of breath with hearts pounding out of our chests. We got into the car and shut the doors as quietly and gently as possible. I turned the car's engine on but kept all the lights off. I had no idea if he had followed us, called the cops, had dogs, anything like that. I wanted to slam the gas and get out of there as fast as possible, but knew I needed to drive very slowly and carefully. I was driving completely in the dark, in an unfamiliar place, basically in the forest. I navigated as best I could with no lights on and we both exhaled with relief when we finally saw the soft glow of the lights on the main road up ahead.

I have no idea if Jose ever found out it was us staking out his house that night. Maybe he was used to animals or something triggering his security setup and didn't think anything of his lights and cameras activating that night. There's no way he didn't find the smoke grenade I dropped, but he'd have no way to connect it to me at all. I never tried to contact him again and wrote off the experience as another lesson learned. A few years later, when I had just moved my practice back into a physical office for the first time in years, Jose actually sent a postcard advertising his IT business to my new office address. It goes without saying that I did not use his services again.

Stabbed & Shot

Remember a little while ago when I mentioned that the cops were called so many times that the apartment refused to renew my lease? Well, the lease was about to be up and we had nowhere to go. The situation felt dire: my credit was shot, I didn't have enough money to put down several months on a new place to help smooth things over, and most landlords aren't eager to rent to someone who was basically kicked out of their last place.

Enter Jessica, a former distant patient of mine who I would also consider an acquaintance. She was an attorney with an impressive resume for how young she was (she was the typical overachiever: she had been top of her class, was very well-spoken, had experience at prestigious firms and was well-connected locally). Upon hearing about my predicament, she suggested I apply to a high-end apartment complex where she happened to live. I was skeptical that I would get approved, but I didn't have any other options. I filled out the application and dropped it off at the leasing office. I wasn't optimistic that it would work out, but instead of worrying too much or applying to some backup places, I just spent the next week high to put it out of my mind.

I had almost forgotten about the application when I got a phone call from the complex at the end of the week. The leasing manager introduced herself and I braced myself for a rejection. "We're pleased to inform you that we've accepted your application. Do you have time this week to come visit and take a look at the available units?" I was in complete disbelief. I had no idea what Jessica said to them but it worked. I made an appointment with the leasing manager and hung up the phone.

Things seemed perfect; the place was nice, Jessica would be a neighbor, and Aileen and I were in desperate need of a fresh start. This would be the perfect chance to do things differently. I was convinced that the change in habitat would allow me to better myself, beat my drug addictions, put an end to the constant domestic violence between us, and finally provide an appropriate environment for Lorenzo, the last remaining child in our care. Aileen was thrilled to hear that we were approved (why wouldn't she be? It was beautiful, 2000 square feet, and she could continue to live a comfortable life paid for entirely by myself without needing to work or contribute to the household in any way. Her only responsibility would be taking care of baby Lorenzo). Her good mood added to my optimism that we could use the fresh start to completely turn our relationship around and be happy with each other.

Everything had worked out, and I was so relieved that it seemed like things were finally turning around for us. Best of all, the new apartment was incredibly close to where Abbie and Giovanni lived. I was finally about to start getting my life under control, and I was hoping that I could start seeing him again. With the inflated confidence of someone on an ungodly amount of amphetamines (this was going to be the very end of it; as soon as we moved to the new place, I would be clean), I decided to give Abbie a call to let her know the good news and see if I could have a visit with Giovanni soon.

Miraculously, she picked up the call. We hadn't spoken in a long time, so I wasn't entirely sure what to expect. She was cautious but agreed to a visit with Giovanni once I was settled in the new place. Looking back, hearing from me out of the blue probably caused some mixed feelings for her. But it was wonderful for me to hear her voice again, and she made the conversation comfortable despite how insane and toxic to her I had been in recent years. That was just the type of person she was, gracious and forgiving. She knew that who I'd turned into the last couple of years wasn't really *me*. She knew me for 16 years as someone who was relatively stable, sober, and a good person. I think she could tell that all I really wanted was to be that guy again. And for the first time in a long time, I felt like I could maybe be that guy again one day.

*   *   *

The next month, we finally made the big move to the new place. It was expensive, brand new, and gorgeous. It was also huge, and it looked even bigger without all of our stuff unpacked yet. 2000 square feet is bigger than you'd expect, but, to me, the high ceilings and openness felt *right*. It felt like the kind of place where you could really get your life together and do everything the right way. Soon.

Adderall and Other False Prophets

The new place was half an hour away from Buddah's house, but a 30-minute drive is a miniscule price to pay for top tier stuff. I was currently out of both Adderall and cocaine, so I shot him a text. He was usually quick to reply, but I waited a little bit with no response from him. There were always people around at his place, so I decided to just head over there. I sent him another text as I was driving. Still nothing.

When I arrived, I was relieved to see his white Escalade out front. I parked behind him and, just like I always did, went through the main door and down the hallway to his apartment door. I could immediately tell something was off. It was dead silent, which was extremely unusual. I knocked with no response. I waited a few seconds. Still nothing, "Cuz?" I asked. Behind the door, I heard a tense but quiet woman's voice. *He said, cuz.* Then silence for a second before the unmistakable sound of pistol hammers being cocked. Definitely more than one.

The door slammed open and Buddah was there, grabbing my shoulders and shoving me out of the doorway into the hallway. "HOW'D YOU GET IN HERE, CRACKHEAD??" He came at me again, and I backed away towards the front door as quickly as possible. He grabbed me again and threw me out into the street, yelling "FUCKING TWEAKER!" before slamming the front door. I never found out for sure what happened that day. A room full of gang members suddenly wanted to shoot me, so someone probably called me a narc and everyone believed it. What I do know is this: because of our close friendship, Buddah saved my life that day and I will forever be grateful. He was a real G. I never saw him again, but I did send him a text: *I hope this life is good to you. Take care of yourself.*

But I couldn't spend too long ruminating on the loss of the friendship and the shock of what just happened: I was out of cocaine and needed to find a new source ASAP. I took my hunt for a new dealer to The Electric Co., a club downtown that Aileen and I frequented. A lot of people in our circle hung out there, and everyone that we knew seemed to also know Justin. He was the bartender and was well-known amongst our friends for several things: he was a good dude, he knew *everyone* (he even got along with the feds who would sometimes come to the club and sit at the end of the bar by themselves), and he would always come up with a different unique cocktail for us to enjoy.

Technically, The Electric Co. was a gay bar. But it was the best club in the area. Everyone from drag queens to typical college kids on a night out went there, the music was great, the vibes were always good, people actually danced. Justin could make anyone comfortable and always made sure everyone was having a good time. He could multitask like nobody else, keeping track of like ten orders at a time in his head, effortlessly making any drink you could imagine and remembering everyone's name while having good conversation.

I was sitting at the bar having one of these conversations with him on a Friday night shortly after the incident with Buddah. The crowd and music were loud but I kept my voice low as I explained my current predicament to him. If you're looking for coke, talk to the guy whose friends with everyone: he came through, and the next day I had an eight ball in my hands. It was good shit, and he introduced me directly to his source.

Niki lived very close to me, in the next town over. She was a big dealer in the area and had a large following so she moved tons of product. Unfortunately, she had almost nothing to show for it. She was an alcoholic and a massive gambling addict. Instead of living the glamorous lifestyle you'd expect of a coke dealer pulling in $4,000.00-$5000.00 a day in cash, she couldn't even cover her rent (once again, addiction makes us behave in self-sabotaging ways that are completely mind-boggling to an outsider). Despite her issues, Niki was never out of stock and she always answered my calls. With a new, reliable supplier in my circle, my big plans of getting clean and making the right choices fell by the wayside.

*   *   *

The date that Abbie and I had set for my visit with Giovanni crept up on me, and it was finally here. I had mixed feelings leading up to the outing. I was excited to finally see Abbie again after everything had transpired. I wanted to see how she was doing. I was apprehensive and nervous to see Giovanni after so much time had passed. He was 3 or 4, old enough to be talking, and I wondered what he would call me.

We met at a nearby park. Even though I was high, I felt a feeling of warmth come over me when I spotted Abbie taking Giovanni out of his car seat from across the parking lot. I crossed the lot to meet up with them. Abbie's friendly greeting almost felt foreign to me; everyone I was surrounded with was corrupt in some way. Nonetheless, it put me at ease. I wore a mask as an extra precaution, ostensibly because of COVID but really to hide as much of my face as possible so it was less obvious that I was fucked up.

The beginning of the visit was wonderful. I played with Giovanni as Abbie and I caught up a little bit. I had forgotten how safe she made me feel. It was the exact same feeling I had in college, when she entered my life for the first time and rescued me when I was drowning in mental illness. After an hour or so, Giovanni became cranky and soon he was crying. He ran to Abbie with his arms up, and that's when I heard another man's name come out of his mouth. He was looking for comfort, and it wasn't from me. Hearing Giovanni asking for Abbie's boyfriend was the most pain I had felt in a long time.

Abbie and I made awkward eye contact. I didn't know what to say; I mumbled "we'll do this again soon" before immediately bolting for the parking lot. I was overcome with emotion as soon as I got into my car and couldn't stop sobbing. It felt like the weight of every choice that led me to this point was on me at once, crushing me. I needed to make the pain stop. I peeled out of the parking lot and sped home, knowing that relief from facing these feelings was waiting for me there, ready to be chopped up with a credit card and snorted directly into my brain.

*   *   *

Before long, Nathan ended up living with me again at the new apartment. One day he just showed up to work at my apartment and never left. He was staying in the second bedroom. We originally had it set up in case the kids were allowed to come for a visit, but CPS had yet to allow that. Nathan's presence always made Aileen more violent; she never liked him living with us and decided to do something about it.

Aileen was in the master bathroom, and Nathan and I were working in the other room. Suddenly, she started banging on the door and walls of the bathroom and screaming that I had locked her in there. The bathroom door only locked from the inside, so I both had no way of locking her in there and no way of opening the door now. My futile attempts to open the locked door just got her increasingly angry.

Before I could think, the corner of our thick, tempered-glass bathroom scale shot through the lightweight bathroom door. She pulled the scale back in the bathroom with her before slamming it again into the hole. She slammed the scale into the door over and over again, the hole in the door expanding with each hit. I caught a glimpse of her face through the hole for a brief second. Her eyes had completely changed color; the sociopathic green/silver flash was in full affect.

Nathan and I ran for the second bedroom as Aileen continued gouging a hole in the door big enough for her to crawl out of. As soon as we were inside, we locked the door and abutted it with a bookcase. Nathan was no stranger to Aileen's violence, and he knew how inhumanly strong she became when she was angry.

For a second, we didn't hear anything. This is usually a bad sign with Aileen, and this time was no different. We were both putting all our weight against the bookshelf to keep the door shut. Suddenly, a heavy wrench shattered the door, missing my head by a few inches. She pulled the wrench out and I caught another glimpse of the look on her face. It was exactly like that scene from *The Shining*, when old Jack axes his way through while smiling the whole time, except she wasn't possessed by a ghost.

Desperate for the crisis to end, Nathan and I called the cops. As usual, she had worn herself out by the time they got there and was casually scrolling on her phone like nothing had happened. I didn't press charges, but the cops did take a look at the door and determined that it was working properly and could only be locked from the inside. The cops left and life continued on. Add another police report to the growing pile.

Soon after, the violence escalated to new heights. One night, we ended up in an argument, no surprise there. It wasn't particularly egregious; just a typical argument for us, I can't even remember the particulars of what set her off. Something snapped inside her and she picked up a loaded 1956 bolt action rifle and waved it in my face. I froze and before I knew it she had grabbed a 4-inch knife off the counter, swung it around, and buried the entire blade in my hip. Before I could even process what had happened, she slammed her palm into my face and broke my nose. I was stunned. I fell to the ground, and she finally left the room after curb-stomping my stomach.

I tended to the damage as best I could. The knife had been freshly sharpened, which prevented a terrible situation from being even worse. I pulled it out, cleaned out the wound and butterflied it. Then I reset my nose. The entire time I was putting myself together, I had one ear out listening for any sign of what she was doing or what state she was in. Somehow, she was calm after all that.

We needed to get out of the house after that, so we took a bunch of coke and went to the casino. It wasn't the most logical choice, but it's what we did. Shortly after arriving, Jessica called my cell phone. She had originally called to ask me for something, but she could hear in my voice that something was very wrong. With Aileen out of earshot, I explained to Jessica that Aileen stabbed me.

"She *stabbed* you?!" Jessica screeched in disbelief. I told her I didn't want to get the cops involved at all and I didn't want Aileen to get into trouble. Jessica was usually the one telling us to avoid contact with law enforcement at all costs for the sake of our CPS case, but she was insistent. I pleaded with her not to say anything. She finally agreed to not call the cops, but she said she wanted to write everything down for her own records. It didn't make much sense to me, but she was a lawyer, so I assumed she knew what she was talking about. She just needed one thing from me and that would be the end of it and asked me to just swing by her apartment complex for a few minutes.

I left Aileen at the casino; it was a short drive from our apartment and I thought Jessica's request would be quick. When I got home, there were detectives waiting to interview me about what had transpired. Jessica lied. I was pissed but told the truth. The detectives took pictures of my wounds and said that everything in the story lined up. I insisted I didn't want to press charges, but what she did to me was so serious they had no choice but to issue an arrest warrant for Aileen.

I returned to the casino but didn't tell Aileen about anything that had just happened. We spent the rest of the day at the casino before it was time to go home. We approached the apartment complex and I entered the parking garage using the private entrance. I parked the car and immediately saw movement out of the corner of my eye. Cops started pouring out of the stairwell. I said nothing, and I could tell Aileen didn't see them. She got out of the car like nothing was wrong and the cops descended on her like vultures on a corpse. Before we could even exchange words, she was being taken away in the back of a squad car. After she left, one of the last remaining cops looked me in the eye before getting into his vehicle. "Someone like her, you can wake up with a knife in your chest or belly. Something to think about."

She spent a few days in jail. I bailed her out. I wish I had a clean explanation for why I don't. There's no logic here, just another turn in the cycle I couldn't seem to break. Abusive, codependent, drug-fueled relationships work like that: you feel tethered to someone even when they're poisoning you. The chaos itself becomes addictive. Aileen was my dopamine spike. I didn't love her, and that was the point, love meant risk, vulnerability, pain. With her, the absence of true emotion felt safer than the weight of my real grief. That's the same reason I stayed numb on drugs 24/7: if I let myself feel, the guilt and loss of Abbie, Giovanni, and everything else I'd destroyed would have consumed me.

The whole episode fizzled out anyway. Aileen was never charged, never did more time. Jessica—our neighbor and conveniently a lawyer—made it vanish, the way she always did. CPS took note, but that was the worst of it. Jessica was everywhere in the storm between Aileen and me: drafting paperwork, offering free legal advice, constantly inserting herself under the guise of "helping us look better for CPS." What I didn't realize until later was how often she enabled Aileen's abuse, sweeping it under the rug and keeping me dependent on her. She never billed me, but her generosity always seemed to flow more freely after I'd sent her prescriptions to the pharmacy.

Soon she was encouraging us to get married, another move, she said, that would help our CPS case. Within weeks, sleep-deprived and high, I was standing in the kitchen in front of a laptop while an ordained minister pronounced Aileen and me husband and wife over Zoom. I gave Niki $3,000.00 to secure a penthouse suite at the casino for the reception. We looked the part, Aileen in a gown, me in a tux, Justin and Nathan at my side as groomsmen, but the real centerpiece of the night wasn't love, it was cocaine. Every surface of that suite was covered with it.

Adderall and Other False Prophets

I remember feeling, in that moment, strangely happy, believing this chaos was somehow good. Looking back with clarity, I see how grotesque it was. That night wasn't a celebration of love, but a parody of it, a dark inversion of the wedding I'd had with Abbie twelve years earlier. Then, I had bound myself to love. Now, I was binding myself to a snake that would coil tighter and tighter until I could barely breathe.

Aces Bay & Tom O'Shea

I needed to be working on a project at all times to keep me busy and sane, and Justin and I were working on a big one during the spring and summer of 2021. We were going to put together a prestigious medical cannabis company and open dispensaries at a time when obtaining a license from the state to do so took an act of God (or just knowing the right person). I had already started a company from scratch, IP and all, that had blossomed into a $30+ million corporation, so why would this be any different? The market was hot, the number of licenses granted by the state was limited, and we were looking to take this idea to the top. Aces Bay Inc, we called it.

We had a lot of smart people at the helm with Justin, in particular, as the standout. He came from a family of great wealth and merit. Heir to the throne of Ford Europe, Justin had not only the name and wealth, but the intelligence to back it up. I was the medical guy (I had already been prescribing medical marijuana for a while at that point). Nathan was our IT god, if you will. Justin brought in a friend of his who had worked in administration at an existing marijuana dispensary. But we needed one more member, someone with an infinite knowledge of growing cannabis. I decided to bring in Tom, a well-known street dealer and grower in the area who had spent years growing and cultivating marijuana.

I had known Tom for many years as a friend of Aileen's. Just like myself, Tom loved the strip club scene. Every now and then he would get me cocaine, although he usually stuck to the drugs that grow out of the ground (weed, mushrooms, etc.). With Aces Bay, he would be our "chief marijuana officer" and we expected him to take the role seriously. However, none of us knew that Tom had been in trouble with the law several times and was actually on the run from a warrant issued due to failure to appear in court out of Kentucky. I should have suspected that he was no stranger to the law when he was able to obtain completely clean urine for me when I needed to pass a drug screen CPS sprung on me with little notice (and trust me, there was no way the piss came from him). Nevertheless, we brought Tom on as our fifth officer and we felt the team was complete.

Adderall and Other False Prophets

We met many times that summer to work on the company, trying to put something tangible together that we could present to investors while doing lots of drugs. On one particular evening, we met at my place and we had more drugs than usual: a ton of stomped coke, molly, ecstasy pills, and God knows what else. Tom thought it would be a good idea to grind everything into a fine powder, mix it all together, and start inhaling massive quantities of this concoction. Nobody in attendance was a stranger to drugs or even sober at that moment, but we were all trying to discuss business and Tom's level of intoxication became distracting and made us uncomfortable. His eyes were red and squinting and his behavior became inappropriate. We all looked at each other and tried to continue with our meeting, but it was clear that Tom needed a bed and possibly a toilet. The meeting ended early and we sent Tom home in an Uber (I over-tipped the driver as a preemptive apology for having to deal with someone in that state). We wrote that night off as hopefully a one-time occurrence, blaming it on Tom's lack of professional experience.

Despite the small hiccups here and there, we thought Aces Bay was off to a great start. The idea was great, and we all believed in it and were dedicated to growing it into something special. Justin and his friend had used their connections to secure a meeting with state legislators. Even though the meeting would take place over the phone, the four of us made the decision to refrain from inviting Tom, just in case he was having another 'off' day. The licensing component would make or break us, and we were competing with companies that were much bigger and more organized. We needed to make a great first impression and couldn't take any chances.

We met a few times without Tom to prepare for the call. Without him, the meetings went smoother and we were a lot more productive. He was still an integral part of the team but didn't need to be involved with every single aspect of the company. He was really kind of a hippie anyway and didn't seem to be as concerned with the functional day-to-day stuff as the rest of us were. The day of the important call drew closer, and the four of us were filled with anticipation. It seemed like we were prepared; I knew I could answer any medical questions that came up on the call. Again, I wasn't a business expert, but it seemed like Justin had a good handle on the logistical stuff every time we met. Things felt good.

The only problems were that we were all high and delusional to a degree, and we didn't recognize the massive hole in the team. Justin had the pedigree and intelligence, but his only real business experience was running a bar. We assumed this would be enough for the time being and planned to bring on a business expert once we got off the ground. This proved to be a mistake; a few minutes into the extremely important call, Justin asked the four legislators for advice on exactly how we should build and structure the company. When I heard those words come out of his mouth, I just about died. We were supposed to bring the schematics to them, not the other way around. The legislators were polite, and the call continued. Justin handled all of the talking, but it soon became clear that he actually had no clue what he was doing. We didn't have a rough business plan, for fuck's sake! Even Aileen overheard the call and got embarrassed, and she knew nothing of actual business.

This seemed like a minor setback, and we tried to take a positive view. At least now we knew our weaknesses and could use that to improve. If anything, the disastrous call only made me more determined to get Aces Bay up and running. We continued meeting, and since it was now obvious that Tom wasn't the major weak point among us, we always invited him. Work continued uneventfully for a week or two and we met as often as we could.

One night, everyone showed up to work except Tom. This was out of character for him and we immediately became concerned. He wasn't answering our calls or texts, and all we could think about was how increasingly erratic he'd been lately (and considering we were all on drugs, that was really saying something). We decided to go check on him. Dressed in the new Aces Bay polo shirts we had ordered to look more legitimate; we took a ride over to the house where Tom was staying. We assumed he might have been high and simply forgotten the meeting, and we planned to continue working from his place if necessary.

As soon as we arrived, it was clear he was not okay. Things were a mess, and he was so smashed we could tell he had been drinking all day. The tone of the visit quickly changed from business to real concern. I can't remember who among us was the first to say they were worried about the amount of drugs and alcohol Tom was consuming, but we all agreed and urged him to consider a rehab program. This wasn't even about the business; we were worried about our friend. It seemed like he was wasting away before our eyes.

Somehow, he had found out that he was excluded from the important phone call so when we suggested rehab he immediately believed that it was because we didn't want him in the company anymore. This couldn't have been further from the truth, but we couldn't convince him otherwise. Despite how drunk and high he was, he didn't get loud or belligerent. He listened to us and was open to our concerns, but when we were done sharing our thoughts, he told us that he was resigning from the company, effective immediately.

We left Tom's house that night in a weird, solemn mood. He listened to us, which was the most important thing. But in my heart, I felt the worst as I had known Tom for the longest, 6 years at that point. I knew he had struggled with severe depression and anxiety and always chose to treat it with drugs and alcohol rather than therapy and pharmaceuticals, but I had never seen him this bad. Before we left, I made sure he knew that his decision to leave the company had no effect on our friendship and he could reach out to me any time. We had known each other for long enough that he knew that I meant what I said. Instead of meeting, the four remaining members of the company decided to go our separate ways for the night.

At approximately 1:00 a.m., I received a text from a mutual friend that she had found Tom hanging from the rafters in the living room of that house. The friend was his on-and-off girlfriend; they had been fighting over God knows what and she went to his house looking to bury the hatchet. She knew I was his longest friendship so I was the first person she broke the news to. Tom had left a suicide note, as many do. In the note, he apologized for being a "deadbeat addict". The feeling that went through me, through us all, cannot be described. It was truly one of the worst things that I had ever felt or will ever feel.

I woke Aileen up and told her, since he had been her friend, too. She immediately burst into tears in disbelief. I could tell she had anger at me as she knew the discussion we had with Tom earlier that night. Before she could really start blaming me, my phone rang and I had to go. When Tom's girlfriend texted me with the news, I had mentioned how shocking it was because I had just seen him a few hours earlier. She mentioned this to the police when they asked her for any information she had about anything Tom did or who he saw that day. The cops called the four of us, the last people to see him alive, and asked if they could meet with us for some questions. I immediately got into the car.

When I arrived at the police station, I saw Justin and we just looked at each other in disbelief. They asked us questions both as a group and individually, probably looking for any inconsistencies. They found none, but obviously we all explained the conversation we had with Tom just prior to our departure earlier that evening. Even though they couldn't Judge me, I could see it in their eyes. I couldn't take it and started to get upset right in front of the questioning officer. I explained that I had known Tom for a lot longer than the other guys and that we had been close on-and-off for years, given his lifestyle. Soon, they said they had enough information and sent us home. We told the truth and had done the right thing by being concerned and trying to offer advice, and they could see by his criminal history (previously unknown to us, as I mentioned earlier) that he was troubled. Even though we hadn't committed any crimes that night, I felt for sure that we had caused, or at least contributed to, Tom's death. For hours I alternated between shock, grief, disbelief, and guilt.

Would Tom have killed himself if we had not stopped by earlier that evening and gave him the addict speech, or if I had never brought him into the company? Was he on the verge anyhow and we just tipped the scales? I ask myself these questions today and still have no answer. I still carry with me a very heavy guilt about the whole situation due to how long I had known Tom and how close we were. I know Justin and Nathan felt grief and guilt as well, but to them, Tom was just a fellow addict who had worked with us briefly as someone in the company. To me, Tom was a human being that loved and deserved love just like any of us and, although he made bad choices (just like we all did), he did not deserve to asphyxiate dangling from his living room ceiling.

Ultimately, I am only responsible for trying to alert Tom to the damage he was doing to himself with the life he was living, but I did not push or steer him towards self-termination. Tom had a very long history of drug and alcohol abuse since his early teens and was even emancipated from his parents. In the end, I choose to remember Tom the way I know he would want me to: as a true G, which he was.

* * *

I wish I could say that this was my only personal experience with losing someone to suicide, but unfortunately that isn't the case. I have lost a lot of people on my journey, from best friends from my hometown to girls I was close with to friends I met while using. While anyone can be suicidal, I will tell you that every single person that met an early demise in my life was involved with drugs, alcohol, or both. Those people I am friends with within this universe who lead normal, productive, healthy lives are all still breathing. And I don't think my experience is uncommon: look at the 27 Club. How many of those folks died because of drugs, alcohol, and/or suicide? Often, it's a combination of serious drug abuse, like heroin, along with depressed mood, leading to active or passive suicide (passive suicide is when someone drinks and/or uses drugs so heavily to the point that their body is so frail that it gives out medically, resulting in death). It's easy to question which comes first: did the person turn to drugs because they were already suicidal or did the drugs fuck with their mental state to the point that suicide seemed like the only solution to their struggles? I think it's a combination of both.

Ultimately, the decision to commit suicide is a complex process that rarely comes abruptly. One must come to the point of feeling so helpless and full of despair that suicide is inevitable. Once their mind is made up, it becomes a matter of opportunity to commit the action (and, as we already know, the action is frequently coupled with a mind-altering substance. Being on drugs has never made anyone *more* rational). Here's an example: Kurt Cobain had his best friend purchase him a shotgun shortly before he committed suicide, and his postmortem tox screen came up positive for heroin. He had no doubt thought about ending his life many times before and even had a failed attempt. But it took the combination of a quick out (gunshot) with an altered mental state (heroin on top of an already-depressed mind) to get him to completion.

Lockwood

Tom was likely high on more than just alcohol that night, serious drugs we didn't know about and probably never will, since his tox screen was never made public. For someone already struggling with depression, that's a dangerous mix. I'm convinced that's what happened, and our conversation may have only reinforced the decision he had already made to end his life.

If there's one thing I wish I could go back and make Tom understand, it's this: even in the darkest, most hopeless moments, when suicide feels like the only escape, things do change. Not as a possibility, but as a certainty. The brain's chemistry never stays fixed; neurotransmitters shift, moods evolve, and what feels unbearable today can ease tomorrow. Depression may turn into anxiety, or quiet into calm, but somewhere along the way there are stretches of balance and peace. Every morning you choose to wake up, there's a chance the chemistry tips in your favor, the day your mind pushes you toward hope, toward help. Nothing lasts forever, except suicide.

A Beacon in the Darkness

Despite the promising start, Aces Bay fizzled out before it could really get off the ground. It didn't feel right to continue without Tom. Looking back, the company was basically doomed from the start, anyway: we may have had an impressive mix of credentials and experience between us, but the company's Achilles' heel was definitely the absence of a seasoned MBA. None of us knew how to even write a business plan, so the structure just wasn't there. At the time, we didn't realize just how much we didn't know. In addition, everyone in the group had a crazy schedule and, as I mentioned earlier, most of us had a drug problem to some degree. Even with proper leadership, it would have been difficult for everything to come together. Tom's suicide was the final nail in the coffin; after that, the enthusiasm just wasn't there.

Even without Aces Bay to focus on, I was still busy. I'm sure you've caught onto the pattern by now, but the beautiful apartment complex in Southfield let us know they would not be renewing our lease. Before we were set to move out, I did a ton of repairs to minimize the damage as best I could (including replacing several doors that Aileen had destroyed). The place was such a wreck that they charged $2181.00 and kept the security deposit. Once again, I was doing a last-minute scramble to try and find a place for Aileen and I to live.

I got lucky the year before with Jessica's personal reference, but that wasn't happening again. There were so many red flags on my rental history that an apartment complex was out of the question. I wasn't sure where to go from here, so I asked someone in the real estate business. Marie was a former patient of mine, a great person and real estate broker. When I told her I was in the market for a private rental, she jumped at the chance to help me find a place. I left out a lot of the details (i.e., that Aileen and I couldn't stop getting kicked out of apartments) and just said that I was in the market to rent privately.

It turns out many private landlords don't bother checking rental history or credit when you can show strong cash flow. I submitted bank statements reflecting $20,000 in monthly income and was quickly approved for a duplex in Bergen, a nice town just next to Southfield. We were set to move in on September 1, 2021. By then,

I had fallen into a pattern, since every lease I signed was only for a year and never renewed, each September seemed to find me packing for yet another move.

With housing secured, I was free to focus all of my time and energy on trying to build my practice into an empire again. Nathan's place acted as the perfect headquarters for this: the house was huge and completely empty except for things like whiteboards, monitors, tons of computers, and other nerd shit. And without Aileen around trying to extract attention from me by force, I could call my patients in peace. After I took care of the day's appointments, Nathan and I would blow some lines and attempt to get some work done. In reality, we would talk nonstop for hours on end (that's just what happens when two people are juiced on uppers. If you've been there, you know what I mean).

Our latest project was an effort to repair my practice's online reputation, which had been damaged after vengeful drug seekers flooded review sites with negativity when I refused to prescribe controlled substances. I brought Nathan in to help, and he recruited some of his friends to post positive reviews in order to bury the bad ones. Soon enough, the good reviews began rolling in, and my online ranking started to rebound. The campaign was working. In truth, I didn't really need it—my patients valued my work and often left genuine reviews on their own. I was simply being impatient.

Even though they were all five stars, most of these recruited reviews were pretty low-effort and sparse. But there was one in particular that stood out to me. It was persuasive and made me look great with specific details that could sway a prospective patient to make an appointment. It didn't sound fake at all, either; it just read like a genuine positive review from someone who had a way with words. It was the kind of review every business owner loves to get. It didn't seem like something that came from one of Nathan's friends and it got my attention. Curious, I asked him who had left it.

Nathan started telling me about Elle. I was expecting him to tell me about some shady miscreant or meth head nerd but quickly tuned back in when I realized this was different. He had met Elle in passing six or seven years before through her ex-husband. After the breakup, the ex-husband showed up drunk to Nathan's old apartment to ask for a bunch of sketchy favors: he wanted to spy on Elle by having Nathan hack into her phone and accounts, and he tried to buy drugs by openly saying he was going to use them to dose a girl (clearly, this dude was a real gentleman). Nathan said no, and the ex-started to get aggressive before suddenly noticing the AK-47 casually leaning against the living room wall (Oh yeah, Nathan knew how to assemble guns from scratch and was studying how to build ghost guns). Like the coward and the bitch, he was, he fled, and Nathan never heard from him again.

Even though they had only met once, Nathan reached out to Elle on social media to warn her about the kind of stuff her ex was seeking out. She thanked him, and they had a brief conversation about the software company she worked for at the time. Years went by without any contact between them until Nathan recently reactivated his social media page, saw her profile, and shot her a message. He recruited her to write a review for me and she agreed. It turned out that it wasn't even technically a fake review she had left; I later found out that she had actually been a patient of another provider at my practice I ran years ago before I moved to California.

Nathan seemed to have a crush on Elle, though he never admitted it outright. What he did say, over and over, was how smart she was, what a great person she was, and how she lived a straight-edge lifestyle. I took it all with a grain of salt. Even high and half sleep-deprived, I could read between the lines, Nathan liked her. He kept bringing her up, and I kept tuning him out, until one detail snapped me to attention. Elle's entire team at work had just been laid off, and she was now looking for job leads. She had spent a few years in the tech world, but constant acquisitions and outsourcing had worn her down. She was ready for something different.

The timing was perfect. I currently had no one answering the phones and doing all the clerical stuff (my last receptionist was Niki, who worked out of my place for a few months in the spring. I caught her drinking almost an entire liter of vodka from my fridge, which seemed to have absolutely no effect on her. I tried to get her to understand how dangerous a situation she was in with her drinking, but she wasn't looking for advice. We amicably parted ways). I asked Aileen to help, but she just ignored the phone all day until the voicemail got full. I had a website where patients could schedule and pay for their own appointments, but it wasn't sustainable to rely only on that. Without someone manning the phone and reception email, current patients couldn't get a hold of the practice for questions and requests, and I was missing out on acquiring the new patients who were trying to book. Not knowing her I asked Nathan if Elle might be interested.

A few days later, Elle showed up at Nathan's house to discuss the job. The meeting was pretty uneventful. Elle was kind of cute but nothing about her really stuck out to me at the time. Nathan and I were high and hadn't slept in days, but she didn't acknowledge it. Our interaction was brief but professional. The job was hers, and I gave her my phone number so we could arrange a time for me to hand off the phone, office Chromebook, and other important work materials to her. She left and Nathan and I resumed working.

The next morning, I finally went home, I had to pick up Aileen for a dentist appointment. What turned out to be a simple errand became an extraordinary coincidence that spared me from another brush with the law. While I was away from Nathan's house for the first time in days, law enforcement descended on the property. Police and FBI agents surrounded it from every side, a helicopter circled overhead, and the entire street was shut down. Nathan woke to the sound of authorities threatening to break down the door if he didn't surrender. Likely, still a little high and completely disoriented, he panicked and grabbed a 1956 bolt-action rifle, presumably in self-defense. What followed was a tense 60-minute standoff, ending only when an FBI negotiator convinced him to come out peacefully. Nathan was arrested on the spot and brought to interrogation. A trifecta of encryption on all his hardware however gave him leverage in the days to come.

I had no idea that all this was going on until later, when he called me from the police department. The initial arrest was for trespassing; it turns out that the scheme he was involved with to take ownership of "abandoned" houses was not a secret loophole and was actually very illegal. The guy who used to live there moved to Florida, but he recently came up to visit and decided to drive by his old house. He knew it hadn't sold and was fully expecting it to be unoccupied, so when he saw the lawn was mowed and the lights were on, he called the cops. Somehow, before an arrest was made, the authorities found evidence that Nathan was also doing things on the dark web that could have been shady (hence why they didn't just send local cops; it looked like someone was not only trespassing but using the property as a homebase to potentially commit other crimes). The rifle plus all of the triple encrypted hard drives the authorities found in the house seemed to confirm their suspicions, and Nathan was being held with a bail set at $10,000.00. (For the record the FBI couldn't crack Nathan's encryption which much later landed him a job with them).

Nathan's arrest coincided with the move from my apartment in Southfield to the new duplex, so I was preoccupied with packing and moving. Meanwhile, I still needed to meet with Elle to give her all the office stuff so the phone could start getting answered again. She had already reached out a few times, but I was a combination of busy and high so it was a little while before I actually replied. I couldn't tell if she was taking this very seriously or was just desperate. I finally gave her a date and time to meet me at a local coffee shop.

She showed up to the coffee shop in office clothes, dress pants and a blouse. We sat down and I started going over everything with her, how scheduling and payments worked, the different appointment types, how to check and send faxes, responding to appointment requests submitted online, the various types of calls and emails we received. It seemed like she was picking everything up, and I was relieved to finally have someone else on board to deal with the administrative stuff. At that point, I was happy just to have a warm body to answer the phone. Anything beyond that was an added bonus and, my gut feeling was that she was a huge bonus.

*   *   *

For the first couple of weeks, Elle worked from her house and I worked from the new duplex (I was still running the practice as telehealth-only due to COVID). About midway through September, I awoke one day to find the internet down. I asked Elle to find and book a coworking space for the day and requested that she join me. It was easier for me to work with someone in person, and I wanted to see for myself how she was running things so far. Patients had complimented her to me, but I also knew they were just happy to have *anyone* answering the phone at that point.

The day was a success. I was impressed with how organized and professional she was, and we worked very well together. Even though I was high, I stayed on schedule and the day went off without a hitch. For the first time in months, I was able to call every patient on the day's schedule and end the day on time. The change of scenery that the coworking space provided was a nice touch, and we agreed to do it again the next day.

At the end of the week, Elle finally brought up the issue of payment. She had been working for me for three or four weeks at that point and I hadn't yet paid her. The weekend before, we had made plans to meet in the mall parking lot so I could pay her, but Aileen started a fight before I could leave and I never showed up. Elle was polite about it, but I didn't want her to think that I was giving her the run-around. I told her I'd text her later and we could meet up after I hit the ATM, one of my favorite things to do (and likely coupled that withdrawal with an eight ball). I always had money for drugs but not for my employee or family.

At home, I could tell by the way that Aileen was acting that I wasn't going to be leaving the house alone. She was in one of her moods and was clearly itching for a fight, but I was really hoping to get this taken care of before another week passed and I owed Elle even more money. When I explained to Aileen why I needed to leave the house, she reluctantly agreed. She was actually happy that I had hired someone, because it meant that one, I wouldn't try to ask her to answer the phones again, and two I would have to spend less time on logistical work and could therefore give her more attention. I'm sure she hoped that I had hired a homosexual man that could also be her "bestie?"

I finally got Aileen out the door and we went to the ATM. I was almost 45 minutes late to meet Elle by this point. I sent her a text apologizing and letting her know I was almost there. I wondered briefly if it would have been smart to give Elle a heads up that I wasn't alone, but Aileen was right next to me in the front seat and could see my text conversation. I knew a message like that would have set her off and made her think something crazy.

We pulled into the lot and Elle came over to the car. I opened the door and got out, and I saw Elle quickly take notice of my visibly angry passenger. Both Nathan and I had briefly mentioned to her how crazy and volatile Aileen was, so she tried to get ahead of any potential drama. She ignored me and immediately introduced herself to Aileen as a sign of respect, only to be met with silence. It had been a smart idea, but it wasn't enough.

Aileen wanted a fight, and she had been expecting Elle to call us out for showing up late so she could escalate the situation. When that didn't happen, she got pissed at me. I had barely handed over the envelope of money to Elle when Aileen jumped into the driver's seat and sped off towards the road, tires squealing. Instead of pulling out and driving away, she turned around in the road and ripped back through the parking lot towards me before screeching to a stop and screaming at me through the window.

I quickly apologized and told Elle that I had to go. She nodded in understanding and I got in the car before Aileen decided to leave without me for real. Even though we had warned Elle about how crazy things were, I knew how jarring it was to see it first-hand and I hoped the drama wouldn't scare her off.

On the ride home, I was pissed and I told Aileen that she had completely embarrassed herself and totally crossed a line by acting out while I was taking care of something for the business. She was annoyed and kept emphasizing that it was late and she wanted to go home. I waited to see if she would have anything nasty to say about Elle, but she didn't.

Despite the dramatic end to the evening, I was glad that they had finally met and that Elle was able to keep her cool. It was a good sign that she wasn't easily pushed into reacting and that Aileen didn't immediately hate her. Aileen knew how to make my life miserable, so her approval of my new staff member was everything. Aileen had somewhat tested Elle in that parking lot for which she "passed" with flying colors.

Under Elle's Spell

Elle wasn't scared off by the outburst, and we kept meeting at the coworking space the next week. Things were running smoothly and Aileen was happy that I was coming home early with the entire day's work wrapped up, with nothing to take my attention off of her. But by the end of the week, she started to get bored at home all day and wanted to tag along to the coworking space.

She seemed to be in a good mood, but I wasn't sure what to expect. Sure, she had every reason to be happy lately: her two biggest needs, money and attention, were being fulfilled. Elle was great at booking new patients and keeping the day on track so money was consistently pouring in, and Nathan's arrest meant that I no longer had a place to escape to when Aileen turned up the heat. But I knew that she could never stay content for long and wondered if she planned to sabotage things in some way.

Surprisingly, things went well and Aileen behaved herself. No reference was made to the parking lot drama from the week before, and the girls got along. Shockingly, Aileen seemed to like Elle. They chatted in between calls and Aileen seemed satisfied that everything was professional between us. I think it definitely helped that she was able to see Elle in broad daylight and realize that she was clearly not a threat: she was brunette, a dork, and petite with no visible curves, which Aileen knew was not 'my type'. Given Aileen's carriage at the time, one would have thought Elle to be completely off my radar. But she wasn't.

When it was time to wrap things up for the day, Aileen seemed almost disappointed. It seemed like they had really gotten along and she was reluctant to say goodbye to Elle for the weekend. On the ride home, Aileen and I agreed that Elle should just come to our house to work going forward instead of me spending the money for the coworking space. Elle agreed and arrived bright and early on Monday morning.

*   *   *

Adderall and Other False Prophets

Things continued peacefully for the next several weeks. Elle worked from the basement and I would call patients from the upstairs bedroom, usually joining her during the lunch hour to brainstorm ideas for how to expand the practice and make it even better. It had been ages since Aileen had allowed me to work this peacefully, and, for the first time in forever, I began each workday without the bullshit of the previous day's missed appointments hanging over my head.

Elle was careful to divide her attention between the two of us, knowing that her "friendship" with Aileen was the key to things running smoothly. They had absolutely nothing in common, but Aileen loved to talk about herself, so there was never a lull in the conversation between them. All Elle had to do was smile and nod, and Aileen was convinced that they were best friends.

In the middle of October, we suddenly heard from Nathan. I had been avoiding his calls for the past few weeks after spending way too much on the inmate phone system. I knew all the calls were monitored and also started to get paranoid after he came dangerously close to saying stupid things about our drug use a couple of times. This time, however, he had big news: his public defender was able to secure his release after meeting with the NSA and he wondered if someone could pick him up on Thursday.

I was relieved. Despite how reluctant I had been to get too involved while he was in jail lest I bring suspicion to myself, I really had been worried about him. I was also eager to continue working on the projects we started before his arrest. He would also need a place to crash (the government had obviously taken control of the abandoned house as part of the arrest), so I started making up the basement in preparation for his arrival. Yes, history continues to repeat itself.

Needless to say, Aileen was not thrilled with this development. She was fed up with the constant pattern of Nathan always ending up at our place and had assumed that his arrest meant that he was out of our hair for good. Nathan's return would inevitably lead to the return of increased drug use for me and a decrease in the amount of attention I could give her. I assured her that it was only temporary and hoped that her newfound friendship with Elle would continue to keep her happy.

By the end of the week, Nathan was fully settled into the basement. We split an eight ball to celebrate, and I set him up with a computer and phone so we could get to work. He started hatching a plan to pay off the several years of delinquent taxes I owed by purchasing stuff on the dark web. I was completely unfamiliar with this stuff and on drugs, so his explanation sounded reasonable to me. Aileen left us alone to work that entire weekend. She was preoccupied with preparing for an upcoming trip to Miami with her sister, who was going to get breast implants.

When Elle showed up on Monday morning, Nathan's work ground to a halt. Her presence was a major distraction for him and he seemed completely oblivious of the fact that she was there to work. Between all of the stimulants and his stupid crush on her, he couldn't stop talking. I could tell she was trying to be polite at first but he never got the hint and continued with his endless story. She opened her Chromebook and started replying to patient emails from the weekend, giving Nathan a perfunctory *Wow, that's crazy* every couple of minutes without looking up. I'm sure he could have happily rambled at her all day, but I couldn't let this continue. Elle would be turning on the office phone in a few minutes and patients would be calling, so I sent Nathan upstairs with a fake task so we could work in peace.

After about an hour, Elle went upstairs to use the bathroom in between calls from patients. She didn't return right away, and I assumed that either Aileen or Nathan had ambushed her on her way back and dragged her into a conversation. I continued working for several minutes until I finally heard her footsteps on the stairs. Silently, Elle came over to the table. Instead of returning to her spot across the table, she sunk into the chair next to me. She looked like she had just seen a ghost.

"Dude," she whispered in a hiss, looking up towards the direction of the stairs to make sure no one was coming. *"You* need *to get a vasectomy."*

I was baffled. What? Where was this coming from? Prior to this, everything was entirely professional between us. She immediately continued. "On my way back, Aileen started telling me about how you guys used to live in California, the mansion and everything. Then she just casually mentions how she *trapped me into a baby*, on purpose, and lied about being on birth control??? She said it like it was this normal thing and *laughed* about it! I barely even know her. Furthermore, Nathan was right there, she said it in front of him!"

Adderall and Other False Prophets

Even though I knew that's what happened, it was still shocking to me to hear that Aileen was so open about what she had done. Proud of it, even! It was embarrassing, both to herself and to me. I brushed it off and tried to change the subject back to work. Elle went back to her seat, still rattled. A few minutes later, a patient called and she busied herself with the request.

The next week, it was finally time for Aileen to head to the airport. I sent her off and immediately returned to the basement, hoping to take advantage of every uninterrupted second we had to work. The pandemic was winding down and I wanted to finally return to practicing in-person. Elle and I had a lot to do, with several meetings lined up that week to check out potential office spaces.

By this point, Nathan was starting to spend more and more time sleeping, which was great for Elle's productivity but not so great for my taxes. Since his release from jail, I had spent over a thousand dollars on the electronics and prepaid Visa gift cards that he supposedly needed for the project and he had nothing to show for it. Aileen kept nagging me about how long he'd be here and the whole situation was really starting to piss me off.

I was thankfully able to push the anger out of my mind for the week and focus on work. For the most part, things were uneventful. Even though Aileen had mostly been behaving herself recently, her absence still led to a noticeable improvement in my stress levels, quality of sleep, and the atmosphere of the house in general. Nathan's arrival had definitely led to increased tensions in my marriage, and even though things were nowhere as near as bad as they used to be, Aileen was beginning to lash out at me during the workday again. Her vacation came just in time, and I hoped that the week in Miami would be enough to interrupt the behavior before it could become a habit again.

Somehow, just like always, word got around that I was alone for the week. In between sessions with patients, I was deflecting advances from girls left and right. Completely out of the blue, a hot blonde stockbroker I used to flirt with even reached out to invite me to Las Vegas for a few days that week to see the Rolling Stones with her on her birthday. "Come on, pull the trigger." Enticing as it was, I had to decline. The return trip from Vegas would place my arrival back at home at almost exactly the same time as Aileen's arrival home from Miami. It was just too risky. If my flight was delayed even by a few minutes, I took the chance of arriving home after she did. If she found out that I went on a trip behind her back, with a girl, to Las Vegas, of all places, it would surely be the mother of all fights. If she caught me walking through the front door, suitcase in tow, she might have just killed me on the spot.

Despite how much I tried to ignore it, there was another reason for me to be disinterested in the random hookup offers. A week or two earlier, I was coming down the basement stairs to work with Elle when something strange happened. When I was about halfway down the stairs, she looked up at me and I almost stopped dead in my tracks. At that moment, something shifted in me. She looked...*different*. I was struck by how pretty she looked. I tried to remember if she always did her hair and makeup like that or if it was new. She was wearing all black, just like she always did, but maybe her outfit was fancier than usual? Did she always look like this and I just hadn't noticed? I never really paid attention to her looks before, but something about her just really grabbed me that day. When I sat down at the table with her, I could feel nothing except the warmth and safety of her energy.

The sudden realization that I was developing feelings for her hit me like a punch in the face, taking me completely by surprise and knocking me off balance. I had to put a stop to the feelings before they intensified; there were about a hundred reasons why it would never work out between us. We were both in relationships, I was ten years her senior, Aileen would have set the house on fire with me in it if she ever found out, and, last but not least, *we worked together*. Everything had been very professional so far (as much as it could be with my obvious drug use and Aileen's constant willingness to fight and argue with me in front of Elle) and I wanted to keep it that way. By that point, she had become such an indispensable asset to the practice that I couldn't risk losing her by expressing feelings that I had every reason to believe she didn't reciprocate. Most of all, falling in love with Elle made me feel extremely vulnerable. I hated the feeling of vulnerability and knew I had to do everything in my power to lock it down.

Fortunately, my life was so busy that it was easy to make myself believe I was adequately suppressing the emotions. CPS was keeping us busy with home visits, family court hearings, and endless mandatory classes (parenting, anger management, domestic violence prevention...). The lease on my Mercedes had ended a few weeks ago, but I hadn't yet returned the vehicle (my credit was now so bad that I knew I would never be approved for a new lease or financing. Once I brought it back, our only transportation would be Aileen's van, which was currently in the shop due to a dangerous electrical problem). Elle and I were busy preparing to open a new in-person office. Jessica had recently pitched me on expanding into aesthetics, so I would also be offering Botox and fillers once the new office opened. This obviously required new training, lots of new procedures to follow, and significant monetary investment. My board certification would need to be renewed soon, and there were dozens of hours of required continuing education I needed to complete before that could happen. Things were hectic, to say the least. Very typical though to try and do everything just because you feel you have the energy to take it all on. Not so much.

As if I wasn't under enough stress, Aileen was beyond fed up with Nathan still living with us and we fought about it constantly. She wasn't wrong to be frustrated: he wasn't paying rent or contributing to the household in any way, and he was a bad influence. I was sick of feeling exhausted every Monday morning after spending another "productive" drug-fueled weekend with him in the basement during which he had actually accomplished nothing. He was always *on the verge* of figuring everything out and I lost track of all the excuses he made for the delay.

We would also be in big trouble with CPS if they caught wind of him living here. At this point, we couldn't afford any more mistakes. If Aileen and I wanted to get the kids back, we needed to follow every demand the agency threw at us and prove how wrong their reports were. Our caseworker needed to leave every home visit convinced that we were completely stable and sober, with no more domestic violence and definitely no random drug addicts living in the house.

Nathan knew how important these visits were. He knew how badly I wanted Lorenzo out of my parents' house and back with us. I couldn't figure out why he wasn't taking this seriously. I would tell him well in advance exactly when our caseworker would be visiting, and he would wait until the last possible second to hide his shit and leave the house. Since the basement was going to be the kids' playroom, the caseworker always included it on her walkthrough and I knew it was only a matter of time before Nathan would get too careless and leave a pocketknife or a rolled-up dollar bill out in the open.

Lockwood

Just like I expected, he fucked up one day and we had a close call that I couldn't forgive. The caseworker showed up a minute or two early for the check-in and Nathan was still in the house. I had to stall and keep her engaged in conversation in the living room while Nathan slipped out of the backdoor. At the end of the visit, Aileen and I exchanged goodbyes with the caseworker and walked her to the front door. I felt my foot brush against something and I looked down to see Nathan's frayed, muddy neon Walmart sneakers with mismatched laces strewn across the floor. I watched in horror as the caseworker looked down at the sneakers, then over to the place where Aileen and I kept our (clean, polished, hole-free) shoes lined up neatly against the wall. The contrast was so stark (and the sneakers so clearly a different size than my shoes) that I knew she could tell they weren't mine. She didn't say anything about the shoes, but she immediately wrapped up the conversation and left.

Anger started to rise inside me. I was fully livid by the time Nathan returned an hour later, barefoot. Since his release from jail, all he did was waste my money, cause fights between me and Aileen, and take up space in the basement. Now, his absolute stupidity was jeopardizing any chance we had of getting the kids back. Why the fuck weren't his shoes in the basement like they were *every single other day*? Was he trying to sabotage us? He probably assumed that as long as we didn't have the kids back, he could keep living here and leeching off of me indefinitely. I think he even liked the fact that he was the reason Aileen and I were fighting so much. Why wouldn't he? The cycle of drama definitely seemed to be working out in his favor: the more Aileen and I fought, the less I wanted to be around her and the more time I spent doing drugs in the basement with Nathan (which, obviously, pissed her off more and led to another fight and more time in the basement).

I gave him an ultimatum: he had three days to complete a simple task or I was kicking him out. I just needed him to log into the router and make the Wi-Fi networks hidden. It was the same thing he always did whenever I moved into a new place; it took him literally thirty seconds. It should have been absolutely no problem for him. Wasn't he the self-proclaimed "IT God," after all?!

He slept for the entire three days and never did what I asked. When he finally woke up, I expected him to pack his things and get out and was shocked to find him wandering around the house like nothing was wrong. After a few minutes, he left to go for a walk. While he was gone, Aileen and I gathered up all of his stuff and put it on the front porch before locking all the doors.

For some reason, Nathan was surprised to see all his shit out front when he got back. He stood on the front porch, peeking through the window and muttering in disbelief. *"C'mon guys, really?"* He obviously hadn't taken my ultimatum seriously, which pissed me off more. I reminded him of my terms and told him that there was an Uber arriving shortly. He asked to speak to Elle, unaware that Aileen was currently in the basement sharing all the gory details that Nathan had verbalized to us about his crush on her. Elle was pretty freaked out and had no desire to engage with Nathan.

He asked if the Uber could take him to another abandoned house that he knew of. I lied and agreed, and he got in the car when it showed up a few minutes later. The destination was actually set to the home of his mother and stepfather; I knew from various conversations with Nathan that they would *not* be happy to see him, but I figured that he was more their responsibility than mine. The car drove away, taking my current biggest problem with it.

One Dose Too Many

After Nathan left, I was able to direct most of my focus on opening the new office with Elle. We printed up flyers and dropped them off at local doctor's offices along with a stack of the new business cards she had designed for me. During this time, we also started viewing potential new office spaces with a commercial real estate broker.

At first, Aileen kept herself busy with a new hobby: hatching and raising chickens. We were heading into winter, so the baby chicks would have to stay indoors for the time being. She transformed the basement space formerly occupied by Nathan into a fenced-in chicken pen, filled with hay and surrounded by heat lamps. I thought this was insane, but it seemed to help her cope with the kids being gone. Elle continued being friendly with Aileen to keep the peace (as long as Aileen was in a good mood, she wasn't as prone to causing the workday fights that led to me missing patient appointments). The "friendship" seemed to be a good influence on Aileen, and she even started trying to dress like Elle. She behaved, for the most part.

A few cracks started to appear in the facade. One day, Elle and I were touring an office for rent when she pulled me aside. Aileen was blowing up her phone with hateful texts, telling her to go home and questioning why we were working on a Friday when I only took patients Monday-Thursday. This came out of absolutely nowhere, and Elle started to worry that she had lost the goodwill with Aileen that she worked so hard to build. We cut the tour short and started heading back to the duplex.

The texts continued to come through, each one more incoherent than the last. By the time we pulled onto my street, they were basically just strings of random letters and I started to get worried. Elle dropped me off in the driveway and went home, figuring it was best to avoid angering Aileen more by coming inside. I went upstairs to find Aileen in bed, unresponsive.

A quick once-over revealed signs of early potential kidney failure and I started to panic. I called 911 and spiked a bag of IV fluids. The following hours were a blur. I was honest and told the EMTs and hospital workers the truth: I had come home after working to find her unresponsive. She had done a ton of drugs the night before, and clearly did the rest during the day. Molly and ecstasy for sure, probably ketamine (my dealer didn't sell it, but she always somehow managed to find it), possibly heroin. She almost had to be intubated.

She was discharged the next day. She had OD'ed, and the whole experience was terrifying and stressful. Even though Aileen admitted that she fucked up, she refused to tell me exactly what other drugs she took besides the MDMA. What if CPS found out about the hospitalization? Or worse, what if she had died? We couldn't continue like this; something needed to change.

By the end of that weekend, I had decided to get sober. This was attempt number 14.5. Drugs caused nothing but chaos in my life, and I needed a change. We both did. We were going to get the kids back, and I was going to run my in-person psych (and aesthetics) practice, clear-headed, well-rested, and eating normally. I set myself up for success by blocking the numbers of everyone I got drugs from and taking a few days off from work after the upcoming weekend to give myself more time to detox. In a few weeks, it would be a brand-new year and I was determined to go into 2022 sober and fully in control.

*　　　*　　　*

As expected, I was exhausted for days as I withdrew from Adderall and cocaine and slept for almost the full five days I had set aside for this very reason. Luckily for me, withdrawal from those two drugs is mainly psychological aside from sleeping a whole bunch initially. I began to gain weight almost immediately and looked visibly healthier. CPS had me take a piss test, and for the first time I wasn't stressed out about whether everything had left my system in time. All of my thoughts made sense, and even Aileen was noticeably less combative. Was this really the secret to all of my problems? Is that all I needed to do?

Things were looking good on the work front, too. The three of us had settled on the perfect office space: close to home, central location near other medical offices, a great reception area, and enough space. There was a room for psychiatric appointments/therapy, a room for the Botox and fillers, and a room for Aileen to do her waxing and facials (she had recently renewed the esthetician license she hadn't used in years and was planning to offer her services at the new office), each with their own locking door. Aileen's approval of the new space was paramount because we were using her name and credit for the lease; while her credit hadn't been great, her financial history was simple and her outstanding debts were a minute fraction of what mine had been. It took only a couple of weeks and a few thousand dollars to get her credit to a place where she would be approved, especially in conjunction with my income.

I finally decided to stop evading the constant calls and letters from Mercedes and do the right thing. I took the plates off my overdue C300 and dropped it off at the dealership late one night, long after closing time. I was so embarrassed that the people I personally knew at Mercedes would see what a mess I had become, but I guess they could probably already tell by the fact I didn't come back at the end of my lease and get a fourth C300. We were now down to only the van between the two of us, and that was a risky prospect. The electrical issue hadn't stopped, and it had burned through three batteries so far in a matter of days. Multiple shops couldn't figure out what was wrong with it.

To help us out, Elle started leaving me with her car and the keys every night so we would have a working vehicle. I would drop her off at her apartment each night and set up an Uber to bring her to work in the morning. This worked out great, but it meant that she would have to stay at our house until 7 or 8 at night if I had a CPS-mandated Zoom group class after work that day.

On one such night, I ended up snapping at her. I was happy with my sobriety, but the novelty had started to wear off and I felt the sudden weight of everything I had to take care of in the near future. The three of us were in the basement after a virtual anger management class, and I started to verbalize a plan that would allow me to get everything done while staying in the good graces of CPS: I wanted to go through a telehealth service and obtain a legitimate script for my ADHD medication, the one and only Dextroamphetamine A.K.A. Adderall.

Elle became alarmed. "Maybe you could get that non-stimulant medication...?" I told her that it didn't work, and it wasn't the first-line treatment anyway, so that was unlikely. The telehealth site was cash-only and specialized in

"ADHD treatment," meaning they slung Adderall scripts at anyone who had the cash. "Well, maybe if you tell them that you're an addict–"

I started to fly into a rage. Being called an addict was always a huge trigger for me, and I mistook her concern as an accusation. I started screaming at Elle, who was completely unprepared for my vitriol and looked stunned. I was so used to being around Aileen, where screaming matches and insults were the norm. But in that moment, I saw nothing but white-hot flashes of anger. "I AM NOT AN ADDICT. *I RUN EMPIRES!*" I finished my tirade and took off upstairs.

After a few minutes, I started to cool off. Aileen came upstairs to tell me that Elle was crying and packing up to go home for the night. I went up to our bedroom on the third floor, feeling like an asshole. It was totally unprofessional and the last thing I wanted to do with so many big things in store for the practice was scare her off. I also didn't want to threaten our friendship; our conversations had gotten deeper and longer since I became sober and I started to look forward to them more and more each day.

Aileen went back downstairs to say goodbye and I heard the front door shut. I was surprised to see that Elle had left her car again for me that night and taken an Uber home. She always took the high road. After my blowup, I was fully expecting her to take her own car. I called her to apologize and was relieved to find her accepting. She apologized, too, but I wanted her to know I was serious. I was always a week or two behind with paying her (sheer forgetfulness, and she was often too polite to remind me), but I recently set up this service that would allow me to directly send her money through my banking app so I was able to bring her current right then and there. I also told her that she could be in charge of designing the new office, picking paint colors and whatnot, and she perked right up. "Oh my God, really? I have so many ideas, it's going to be sick! I'll show you tomorrow," she effused. I also agreed that it was for the best that I refrain from seeking Adderall, to her relief.

The coming weeks were full of promise as everything gradually started to fall into place. We signed the lease for the office and it would be ours on February 1st. Aileen and I scoured Craigslist looking for secondhand furniture for the office and we had some great finds so far. I had a friend who worked at U-Haul, so I got a great deal on a truck to keep the furniture in until we could start moving everything in. Elle was great at tracking down free continuing medical education courses online and I was making slow but steady progress towards the total number of hours I would need to renew my board certification. I attended all the necessary online seminars to learn how to inject Botox and fillers and would soon make a trip to Boston for the two-day in-person part of the course. I went to the bank to update my business account with the new practice address and info and added Elle as an authorized user with her own debit card (this was something I always did when running an in-person practice. I would be way too busy to worry that every last expense was being taken care of, and part of my office manager's job was to make sure everything got paid on time and all receipts were logged).

I started to mention to my patients that the office would be opening soon, and they were thrilled. Many of them had been with me for years and hadn't met with me face-to-face, without a phone or computer screen, since before the pandemic started. The women were excited in particular to hear about my new injectable services, and several offered their faces to me to practice on in exchange for a discount.

In the middle of January, Aileen, Elle, and I got ready to head to Boston for the aesthetic injecting course. A few minutes before we were set to hit the road in Elle's car (the van still couldn't be relied upon to go a few miles, let alone a trip that long), I realized that my debit card was missing. The three of us spent a few minutes looking for it before Elle spoke up. "Well, I have the one you got me, so we can just use that for the trip."

As soon as the words left her mouth, my blood ran cold. She had no reason to expect that her being on my business account would be a problem, but Aileen took it as a massive personal offense. "Oh, so you trust *Elle*, but not me?!"

"Of course, I trust Elle!" I cried. In response, Aileen stomped upstairs, yelling that the trip was off. I took off after her to smooth things over, telling Elle to wait downstairs. I was certain that I could talk Aileen down. If I couldn't, the entire trip would be cancelled and I'd lose thousands of dollars already spent on the hotel and the class. I couldn't go to Boston with just Elle; it would come across as inappropriate and Aileen would have killed me. And I couldn't have asked Elle to lend me her car to take to Boston for the whole weekend without her.

Adderall and Other False Prophets

I pulled out all the stops with Aileen and she ultimately got stoned and acquiesced. She would do that from time to time with the weed, it would cool her off. The three of us made the trip to Boston for the class, sharing one hotel room with two beds. Elle was careful to tread very lightly around Aileen, and I was grateful. Fortunately, the rest of the weekend was uneventful and I returned home with a certificate and some real-life experience in the world of plastics.

Once we got back home, things really started to ramp up. We had less than two weeks until our lease started for the office, and our official opening date was set only a few days after. Elle had gotten everything in place for Internet and insurance at the new office, as well as doing all the research to find the special fridge and log sheets we would need in order to adhere to the regulations around injectables. I opened accounts with suppliers. This was really happening.

While I was confident that I could handle the aesthetics stuff from a technical and safety standpoint, I still worried that I had no idea what I was doing. Aileen had gotten her lip fillers and Botox too recently to go again so I could observe the process. A golden opportunity seemed to present itself when Jessica told me that she had an upcoming appointment. She said that I could come with her, and she would lay the groundwork for me to shadow her provider for a little bit. Score!

Elle waited in her car with Aileen while Jessica and I went into the office for the appointment. None of this really made sense to me, women in their 30s getting stuck in the face with needles to look 'younger'. But it was a massive moneymaker, and it's always good to diversify. So, I introduced myself to the provider, watched, and took mental notes. This wasn't difficult at all.

After the appointment, Jessica pulled me into her car to talk business for a few minutes before asking to meet Elle. Jessica rolled down her window and Elle introduced herself. Considering that it looked like Jessica had just lost a fight with a nest of angry wasps, their introduction seemed to go well. I felt like I had a solid team behind me and I was surer than ever that we'd be a success.

Later in the day, I was heading back when I received a call from Jessica. She told me how she felt like Elle had a "dark energy" and warned me to be very careful with her. This was totally out of left field. I thought their meeting had gone well. Confused, I just thanked her for looking out and we hung up. I was baffled by the cryptic "warning" and put it out of my mind.

*   *   *

The final two weeks before we were set to open went by in a blur. Aileen had me order a few thousand dollars' worth of supplies and furniture for her esthetician's room (including a rug, huge storage shelves and an actual adjustable facial chair), and the packages kept rolling in. I was in talks with the local Chamber of Commerce in order to obtain a listing, and I was faced with everything I still had left to do in such a short time. The pressure was on, and I couldn't afford to waste a minute.

I knew how I could be more productive and ensure everything got done in time: sleep a little bit less and focus a little bit more. I don't think I need to be more explicit than that at this point. Before I could think twice, the deal was done and I had once again traded my sobriety and ability to think clearly in exchange for the little orange pills that were nothing but false prophets. In a perfect world, sure, sobriety would have been great. But this was the real world, and I had shit to take care of.

The next weekend, Aileen and I went to Connecticut for a rare visit with Lorenzo and my parents. I made sure not to take any Adderall that day; the visit was only allowed due to my "sobriety" and my parents could always tell when I was using. The visit was beautiful and I immediately became wracked with guilt. Spending time with Lorenzo and my family and eating the incredible dinner that my mom made me realize that what I really wanted in life was to be healthy and have my family back.

On the car ride home, I admitted to Aileen how I had fucked up. Surprisingly, she wasn't angry at me. No, this was Elle's fault. She had caused my relapse a few days before when she hurriedly slipped a pill into my hand on the way home after hearing how stressed I was about everything I still had left to do.

The next day was Sunday, and I texted Elle to come over for a last-minute work task. Aileen intercepted her at the front door while I pretended to be asleep upstairs, able to hear through the vents every word they exchanged. Aileen was pissed, and I was shocked to hear that Elle lied and denied everything. They went back and forth for about 30 minutes until eventually Aileen accepted the lie and calmed down. Elle came upstairs but left after realizing I was "asleep".

I was still surprised how easily she was able to lie, and for a few minutes I wondered if I had misJudged her character. Before Aileen could start in on me, I rang Elle's phone. "Why did you lie to my wife?"

"*Uh...what?*" Again, with the bullshit. She was secretly on speaker because I assumed if I called her personally, she would acknowledge how she gave me the pill (and maybe even offer more). Instead, she acted confused and denied causing my relapse. I started the call angry, and it sounded like she was starting to cry on the other end. Eventually I softened, explaining what had happened on the trip, my realization, and how bad drugs were for me. I needed to be sober in order to be the best provider, father, husband, boss, and friend that I could be. Aileen made her presence on the call known so she could back me up.

We all got a little emotional, but not in a bad way. The call ended on a high note, with Elle eventually apologizing and affirming that she understood how big of a deal it was. Aileen and I agreed to forgive the misstep and said that Monday would be a fresh start.

Except that isn't how I relapsed. In reality, it was a decision I made for myself. While working in the basement that week, I took one of the Adderall tablets I always kept in my pill organizer for "emergencies" (I always kept a couple pills around whenever I tried to get sober so I didn't start to get anxious and start seeking them out. It was a habit that I picked up back when I smoked cigarettes. I'd always keep one in my desk when trying to quit). I took the pill right in front of Elle, while she was tied up on a phone call with a patient and couldn't try and stop me. Worry spread across her face. After she hung up, she started to anxiously voice her concerns. I dismissed her handwringing with a single question. "Do you wanna get some work done, or not?"

When I told Aileen that Elle gave me the pill that led to me using again, I wasn't trying to throw her under the bus for something that she hadn't actually done. In fact, at the time, I didn't even know I was lying. I think my brain was just trying to shield me from taking responsibility for causing my own relapse. The consequences at home would be less severe if Aileen had someone other than me to blame. And maybe Jessica's "warning" about Elle played a part, too – it was fresh in my mind, perfect for my brain to use when constructing a confabulation. It allowed me to come clean while preserving myself. I'm sure the entire situation was confusing for Elle. Her apology was out of a genuine desire to keep the peace and keep her job.

I wish I could say that this was the end of my mental confabulations and the beginning of lasting sobriety. However, my confession that I was "off the wagon" only led to me giving myself full permission to abuse drugs as heavily as before. With everything "back to normal," I was completely unaware of the insane storm of chaos that would be unleashed on my life in the coming months.

Hallucinations and Handcuffs

The first week in the new office was great, for the most part. The place may have looked a little dated, but Elle had lots of great ideas for making everything look modern and expensive. We spent a few hours one night texting about design plans for the office, making lists of what we would need from Home Depot and Amazon, and planning to get started early the next morning. With a plan in place, we ended the conversation and I decided to get some sleep.

A punch to the face was my wake-up alarm the next morning, followed by a litany of insults. Aileen was pissed, which was starting to happen more and more often these days. We had a good couple of weeks (well, "good" compared to our usual endless fighting, but probably still toxic by normal standards), but she began to act up again when she started to realize that her position as my wife didn't entitle her to everything she was expecting. For example, she insisted on accompanying Elle and I to the office any time she wanted and didn't get why she couldn't blast videos from her iPhone at max volume in the same rooms where Elle and I were on calls with patients. Or she'd get pissed when I would drive the three of us to the office in Elle's car, and Elle didn't immediately think to get into the backseat (of her own car, that she was graciously letting me drive around in the first place) so Aileen could sit in front with me (again, when she would have no reason to even come with us in the first place and would only lead to me being less productive than if she wasn't there).

But this time, I had no idea why she was upset with me. I had been sleeping! I pieced from the screeching rant that she had taken my phone from next to me, used my sleeping face to unlock it, and then went through my texts. When she figured out that the content of all my texts was innocent ("here's a link to a sharps container on Amazon, for the used Botox needles," "it looks like this peel-and-stick fake marble countertop doesn't need a heat gun, awesome"), she decided that she was mad that I was texting "another woman" (Elle) "so late at night" (9:45 p.m.).

Oh, and she was thoughtful enough to send an essay-length text message to Elle for daring to reply to my texts (give me a break, of course she was going to reply to work texts from her boss). As if that wasn't embarrassing enough, Aileen signed off her message with "YOU DO NOT HAVE PUSSY RIGHTS OVER ME" ("pussy rights" or PR meaning how a guy has to put up with constant communication/texting from a girl he's regularly getting pussy from). It was not actually an accusation of cheating (even insane, jealous Aileen could tell everything was platonic and professional), more of a "every second of my husband's time belongs to ME. Therefore, you have stolen a possession of mine and will be punished accordingly" situation. The worst part is that the text conversation between me and Elle never "stole" any of my attention away from Aileen; I only reached out to Elle in the first place because Aileen was busy doing something on her phone, and I figured that having a plan in place beforehand would result in a shorter workday.

We opened it to the public unceremoniously. Even though most patients still chose telehealth at first out of habit, I spent every clinical day (Monday-Thursday) at the office. Aileen's basement chickens were a little older now and had become noisy, and multiple patients heard them during their sessions and asked me about it and the duplex had been the scene of too many fights recently. I needed a clear boundary between home and work to help me focus better. When I came into the office, I could be my real self again – the professional, competent provider that patients looked to as an authority, instead of the drug addict stuck in an abusive marriage stuck at home.

I honestly don't know why I thought that would work. With each passing day, it became clearer that Aileen did not respect the office as a place of business where medical care was provided. To her, it was an extension of our home, a battleground to continue fights that she had started that morning or even the night before. She would make TikTok videos in the waiting area, even if Elle was on a call or patients were waiting. Her interruptions were constant, and she was totally oblivious to how inappropriate her presence was. With more and more patients choosing in-person appointments, my mind was flooded with nightmare scenarios of her potentially barging in while I was mid-session with a patient in my room. She didn't care either, she would do it just for the look on my face or the patient's face.

Her waxing/facial/whatever "business" was going absolutely nowhere. She did nothing to get the word out, so she had a grand total of zero customers and zero desire to change that. Between the expensive furniture and decor, her license renewals, business cards, fancy white esthetician coat with her name embroidered on it, extra cell phone as a "business line," and the fact that we had picked this big of an office specifically to accommodate her endeavor along with the medical stuff, I ended up wasting around $5000.00 on this crap and endless amount of headache. If it wasn't going to keep her occupied and out of my hair, the least she could have done was hang out in her designated room when she insisted on being at the office. I did have female patients who wanted to book with her but she could care less. Just an excuse to be at the office and remain in our daily lives.

With the realization that the office wasn't the safe haven I had looked forward to for months, I leaned further into drugs as a coping mechanism. On Adderall and coke, I was too high or focused to be bothered by Aileen's bullshit. It was like a suit of white armor. But even a suit of armor can get cracked. She could always tell when I was trying to tune out her noise, and she would respond by turning up the volume twice as loud.

A week went by, each day more miserable than the last. First it was that she was sick of spending so much time at the office. Instead of doing the logical thing and staying home, she just came up with a new routine for us. No more Elle coming to pick us up in the morning an hour before we opened the office. Instead, Elle was to open up shop alone. Aileen and I would take an Uber there in time for my first in-person patient of the day (usually in the early afternoon) and take an Uber home after the last in-person. The constant traveling throughout the day ensured that I could never get fully locked into "work mode". Frustrating, annoying, but I figured it was temporary and I would make it work. Then, she told Elle to stop coming to my room to physically deliver messages when I was free. She was to text or email them to me, where they would inevitably languish and get missed (and God forbid I try to catch up at home instead of giving attention to Aileen).

From the second we left the office at night until my first patient the next morning, Aileen did nothing but accost me with vile insults and accusations. If I fell asleep, she would wake me up and try to re-hash an earlier argument, taking my disoriented twilight state as "proof" that my earlier statements on whatever it was were just rehearsed lies. She always knew exactly what to say to cause me the most pain, constantly reminding me that I "abandoned" Giovanni and telling me that I was "neglecting" her just like I did to Abbie (despite the fact that I was giving in to all of her ridiculous demands and spending every second with her). She would never have the quality of attention I had given Abbie.

It was like my original play to take this stripper and her kids and make the perfect family had been turned against me. Something I forgot originally is that these girls were used to guys' games and I doubt I was the first savior case happening in that strip club. She knew it and let me play right into her game and turned it all against me without me seeing it. She played the long game and was very good at it.

Every interaction left me feeling hollower, and smaller, like a stream of water eroding a stone away. On a Wednesday night towards the end of February, she got so angry at me about something that she pulled a knife out of the knife block in the kitchen. It ended up being an empty threat, which pissed me off that she would even play like that.

The next day, I woke up before Aileen and just grabbed an Uber into the office without her. I showed up showered, in my dress clothes, and ready to work at the same time as Elle. "Oh, thank God," she exhaled in relief. "I was afraid I'd be alone here all day again."

I'm assuming that Aileen woke up at around noon that day, because that's when she sent her first text of the day to me, asking where I was. I told her that a patient asked to switch their appointment from virtual to in-person at the last minute, which she seemed to accept. Unsurprisingly, things went smoothly. When it was just me and Elle, I somehow miraculously had not only enough time to stay on top of everything, but to prepare for the coming days as well.

After the last patient, I asked Elle for a ride to the pharmacy, and then we went to Home Depot to finally take care of our list from two weeks ago. Aileen started hammering away at me through texts, and I told her I was running errands for the office and left it at that. Clearly not satisfied with my explanation, she started texting Elle, who sent a picture of me browsing the aisles of Home Depot. It was proof that we were both telling the truth, and Aileen hated the hardware store, anyway. She sent me a huffy text reminding me that we had a virtual anger management class for CPS that night before finally shutting up for a little while.

Adderall and Other False Prophets

I dragged out the shopping trip and, before we knew it, it was time for my class. I ended up taking it on my phone in Elle's car in the Home Depot parking lot. I was attentive and engaged, eagerly participating in the corny conversation the instructor was trying to lead. Aileen was fuming and spent the whole class sending me nasty texts about how I clearly wasn't taking the class seriously since I didn't come home to attend, I was the reason her kids got taken away, etc. (which obviously fell flat; she was the one ignoring the class and trying to fight with me while the instructor was literally in the middle of complimenting my insight).

After the class, Elle drove me to the office parking lot. Instead of getting out immediately and calling an Uber, we hung out a little bit more and started talking. It felt nice, and I realized just how long it had been since our last real conversation. I opened up about how dead I was feeling with Aileen. Elle had obviously witnessed plenty of Aileen's orchestrated chaos, and this wasn't the first time we talked about it. But being away from Aileen for the whole day was freeing, and I spoke with a candor that surprised me.

It was starting to get late, and I knew that the office was the first place Aileen would look if she was trying to track me down. I had the van towed to another mechanic a few days earlier in hopes of finally finding out the issue, so she didn't have access to a vehicle. In a way that was worse, because if she took an Uber to find me, I would have no idea what type of car to look out for. I drove us to a parking lot a few towns over to finish our conversation.

Elle told me that she would have to go home soon, but I didn't want the night to end. I could tell that she didn't, either, and she could definitely tell that I was truly going through some shit. She was lonely and disconnected, sleeping alone on her couch since last July. I presented her with the flimsiest excuse ("Say that you need to sign paperwork for the new office and we need to help Jessica draft it up, and we can only do it tonight, and it will probably take the whole night") and she sent a text home with the news. The night was ours.

I decided to take her to the Velvet Room, but we never made it out of the car. We spoke for hours about everything. I explained that my life wasn't always like this. I told her about my childhood, college, previous jobs, and my marriage to Abbie. I shared some intimate things about myself, things that Aileen loved to throw in my face and insult me for, and Elle was completely unfazed and told me it was normal. It felt like forever since the last time someone actually listened to me. To be understood is an incredible feeling, and it felt like I was glowing. We sat in the front seat of her car until the club was closed and the parking lot was empty.

With the sun finally emerging over the horizon, she told me that she had to stop back home to get her daughter ready for school and take her to the bus stop. It was so different from any responsibilities I had in my life, and I loved feeling like we were doing the right thing. In that moment, everything felt right. I sat in her apartment parking lot until she finally emerged with her 8-year-old daughter, Siobhan.

Siobhan opened the door to the backseat and I turned around to introduce myself as she sat down. Our eyes met, and I will never forget the way that little girl looked at me. I saw an understanding well beyond her years, and it felt like she saw me for who I truly am and accepted me, just as her mother did. We took her to the bus stop, and I tried to plan where to go next.

I told Elle about a car dealership a patient recommended to me. Supposedly they would work with me based on my income and didn't concern themselves with trivial matters like bad credit. They wouldn't open for another hour or two, but I didn't mind having more time to continue our conversation. On the way there, I made a comment about how pissed Aileen was going to be when she figured out that I never came home last night.

"You're allowed to have friends. But more importantly, you have every right to remove yourself from a situation that is violent and dangerous...literally, this is an actual abusive relationship. She's going to kill you." Elle spoke with that inflection young women have where the end of every sentence goes up as if it were a question, but her words were tinged with both sincerity and a somber gravity.

We made it to the dealership, and I parked the car waiting until they opened. Neither of us had said anything since she last spoke, and I was still turning over her words in my mind. Finally, I spoke. "You're right." I asked her to book me a hotel at the casino for the night, using her email so Aileen couldn't find out where I was if she currently had access to my accounts. She pulled out her phone and got to work. I could tell she was drowsy from the all-nighter.

After a few minutes, my phone started vibrating. My dad was calling. I answered, unsure of what to expect (Aileen was fond of "tattling" on me to my parents when she was upset, usually spinning a situation to make me look dangerous and completely off-the-rails and presenting herself as an innocent victim or noble for "putting up" with it). He was just checking in, he knew Friday was my day off, etc. I glanced over at Elle in the passenger seat and asked my dad if he could go get my mom, too.

He put me on speaker and my mom greeted me. I took a deep breath, feeling safe and sure of things, and started to tell them everything about Aileen's abuse. I swept everything out from under the rug. It was cathartic; for so long, I had (unconvincingly) insisted to them that I had everything under control. They obviously knew things were bad and I had a major problem with drugs (CPS had given them custody of Lorenzo, for God's sake), but they seemed to just think that Aileen and I had a run-of-the-mill, mutually toxic relationship. No longer concerned about appearing "weak" or worrying that they would use the information against me, I told them about how she stabbed me, hit me with a hammer, and how she tried to interfere with my work. They were aghast.

I told them about the time I returned from work to find Lorenzo still in his crib, still in the same diaper he was wearing when I left 12 hours earlier. I gave him a bottle of water, and he pounded the entire thing. She was in bed a few feet away, texting on her phone, completely oblivious. I printed out the contact log for our AT&T account. She had spent the entire day texting that politician I mentioned earlier (the one who bought the Christmas gifts for her kids), while our baby went all day without food or water. Aileen's youngest daughter told me that "Mommy leaves Lorenzo in poopy diapers all day".

My mom was sobbing. "*Why didn't you leave her?*"

"I don't know!" I was crying, too. I had been for a while, and Elle put her hand on my shoulder. It was platonic, but it was the first time she ever touched me, and it was calming. I told my parents that I needed to leave her, I was ready, I wanted to raise Lorenzo.

"That's something to aim for," my dad said. "But think of how much time you spend working. Do you have a responsible young lady in your life who would be able to help you raise Lorenzo?"

Again, I looked over at Elle. I had the call on speaker, but I could tell that she was trying to give me as much privacy as possible. "Yeah. I do."

"Well, that's good. That's a start." My dad knew me well enough that he wasn't surprised to hear I was stepping out on Aileen. I meant what I said, and I started to imagine what Elle would be like as a mother to Lorenzo. It just felt *right*.

The phone call ended on a high note. The dealership had opened, but I decided not to go inside. I started to drive towards the casino. Maybe they would let me check in a few hours early. I was full of hope and let myself picture a new life with Elle, overcome with how warm and safe the thought made me feel. She never reacted to what I said to my dad, but she must have heard. The silence between us was so comfortable that I didn't notice the moment when her sleepy half-lidded eyes slipped fully closed.

On the highway, I heard a noise from the passenger seat that snapped me out of my daydreams and into nurse mode. Elle was slumped forward, and it sounded and looked like her airway was blocked. I immediately flew into panic. She must be having a reaction to something. There was nowhere to pull over and we were miles until the next exit. Terrified, I tried to figure out what to do. I imagined every worst-case scenario, starting with the possibility that she was dead and ending with the consequences of being found with my younger, female, dead employee.

I kept my left hand on the steering wheel and reached over with my right hand, lifting her head as far up as possible in an attempt to open her trachea. The occlusion noises stopped. I kept holding her head upwards, just in case, and she eventually opened her eyes, however it felt like hours had gone by.

"Woah. Hi," she said sleepily. I was still leaning towards her halfway across the car, foot almost slipping off the pedal. "What happened? I fell asleep." She could read the terror on my face. I almost started crying again as I told her what happened, how I thought she had stopped breathing and worried she was dead or dying.

Thankfully, she was fine. I was incredibly relieved. We finally pulled into the casino parking garage, and I was never so happy to see her beautiful smile. This is what happens when you stay up all night without the help of uppers, you pass out hard.

*   *   *

I blocked Aileen's number and checked into the hotel. Once in the room, Elle and I tried to get some work done. I opened my laptop to start working on some continuing education credits and tried to come up with some way that I could sneak into the house to get my necessary meds without Aileen noticing. Across the room, Elle was sitting cross-legged on the bed, replying to emails. A couple of hours passed. Without all of the chemical advantages I was currently experiencing, Elle eventually stretched out on the bed and took a nap (fortunately, she stayed breathing the entire time).

At the first hint of darkness in the sky, I shook her awake. She looked around, still half asleep, before picking up her phone and squinting at it. She looked out the window. "Is it a.m. or p.m. right now? How long have I been asleep?"

"Like two hours maybe?" It's Friday night. Let's go back to the Velvet Room, since we never got to go inside last night," I was excited. "To celebrate the first day of the rest of my life."

She agreed, and we tried to clean ourselves up a little bit. We each pounded a Red Bull before heading to the car. The office was on the way to the strip club, so I decided to make a pit stop. We stopped inside and I hooked Elle up to a bag of IV fluid. A jolt of hydration like that would make *anyone* ready to hit the town, and soon she was back to her usual chatty self. I must have had dust in my veins at that point as I was never hydrating myself.

I parked Elle's car at the VR. I could tell by the mix of vehicles in the very full parking lot that the place was bumping and it would be a fun night. We were in the middle of a conversation again, but I was determined to actually make it inside the club that night. I grabbed my wallet and turned off the car. "Wait," I stopped Elle as she went to open her door, my brain concocting a plan in real time. "When we go inside, we should pretend to be together, like as a joke."

Lockwood

Without hesitating or questioning how nonsensical this "plan" was, Elle agreed. We got out of the car and she took my hand in hers as we approached the massive, ornate, infamous red door that led to the Velvet Room. It swung open, and I took in all the familiar sights and sounds of my surrogate home. The bouncers knew me, most of the girls knew me, and the bartenders knew me, especially Molly. And they knew Aileen, too. But they all hated her almost as much as they liked me (and they liked me a lot), so I wasn't worried about anything.

From the minute we made our entrance, I felt like I was floating. I went to pay for the cover and was told to put my wallet away, we were good. I looked over to Molly behind the bar as she smiled back and winked. We walked to a table, and it was almost like the music stopped. I felt like a celebrity on the red carpet, or a quarterback after winning the Super Bowl. I ordered and grabbed our drinks from Molly, who gave me a nod of approval before I returned to the table. She wasn't the type to pry or ask questions, but we knew each other well enough that we cared about each other and she was familiar with my Aileen situation.

I set down our drinks and took my place at the table across from Elle. In between sips, our easy conversation bounced between topics like a bee flitting between flowers. Everything else fell away, and suddenly I was no longer inside a busy club. The only sensory input I was getting was her, the sound of her laugh, the sight of her perched across from me in yesterday's work clothes, the feeling that spread through my body when we were making eye contact. And now, suddenly, the warmth and weight of her body as she crawled up into my lap. "We're supposed to look like we're together, remember?" she explained. I nodded.

We were in our own universe, and we sat like that for a lifetime. She was pressed against my chest, with my arms around her and my chin resting on the top of her head. She was so still that I wondered if she fell asleep. It had been two months since Elle and I locked eyes in the basement and I started to see her in a new light. I couldn't kill the feelings growing within me since then, and now I couldn't ignore them, either. I lowered my voice and told her everything that was on my mind, whether she heard me or not. I wanted this girl to know that I liked her a lot more than she knew, and I think I made that point clear. I was awake, and free, and she made me feel seen. And she made me feel loved for who I really was, not who I pretended to be or my family expected me to be.

I could see Molly from behind the bar again as she smiled back. Molly was what I call an OG without a doubt and actually ran the VR for a more private family business owner out of Boston. I'll just say this, the VR was in a residential area and never ever had police waiting as the drunk customer base emptied out onto the roads from 10:00 p.m.-5:00 a.m. The place was more than meets the eye and a ton of fun. None of the girls came over to us to pimp for tips or dances. There was a blanket of respect and Elle and I at the center. I don't know how long we sat like that that evening. It may have been an hour or the whole night. All I remember was really opening up to her telling her everything I had been thinking regarding the two of us not knowing if she was listening or fast asleep. The ice melted in my still full drink soaking the napkin causing a small pool of water on the table. The only thing I was conscious of was making sure Molly knew that Elle had passed out, not nodded out as many customers would do right there at the bar. Molly knew that I didn't swim in those types of circles, and even if she had nodded out, I was the guy with the most medical training in the building anyhow.

I walked Elle to the car after VR closed and we sat and talked for a while. I remember she had a glow to her, something I hadn't seen in a long time (at least 5 years at that point). I had a deep desire to kiss her but didn't want to initiate. I've kind of been like that my whole life; the girl had initiated the first kiss in most of my relationships. But I didn't want to wait any longer. Fuck it, I leaned in and started making out with her. I could feel her pushing towards me, embracing the moment. We were making out so intensely that I felt like a high schooler again and I was eating it up. It was super hot, but emotional, too. I had to pull back every few minutes to breathlessly repeat my feelings from earlier – *You make me want to live life again. You're a type of beautiful I didn't know existed* – before immediately grabbing her face again and returning to the kiss.

We continued like that for what must have been an hour before we took off back to the hotel. I was ready to do some more drugs and really get the party going. I knew I loved that girl, and I knew I wanted to be with her. I was making it happen. We made it back to the room, and Elle immediately got on the bed. I sat next to her and started caressing her hair and just looking at her fondly as her eyelids got heavier and heavier with exhaustion. I figured she must have been starving, having subsisted on nothing but gas station candy bars and energy drinks this entire time, so I got the bright idea to order room service for her. After wolfing down some chicken parm, she finally passed out. I continued the party alone, blowing so many lines and taking so much Adderall that I almost forgot that I hadn't taken my meds in days and they were still at home with Aileen. *Son of a bitch*, I remember thinking. *Well, I have cocaine, so I should be okay.*

As the night turned into early morning, the room started to look more sinister to me. Paranoia was creeping in, and I became convinced that the FBI agents were huddled outside, waiting to kick the door in. I had drugs on me, and there was a girl in here, passed out. She was short and thin, what if they thought she was underage? Was I being set up? The light on the smoke detector was blinking in a strange way, and I started thinking that it was a camera, streaming everything live to the internet. I was terrified; at this point, they had me in the bag. I grabbed my knife and stood near the door, ready for when they came charging in.

I waited in that position for several hours, but they never came. Holy shit, I was in a bad way. I *needed* my medication. I grabbed Elle's car keys and sprinted through the halls and into the parking garage before hopping in her car and taking off in the direction of the duplex. I figured I could probably get back before Elle woke up.

As soon as I got home, Aileen tried to intercept me for a confrontation. Still paranoid, I pushed past her and ran up the stairs, two at a time. I dove towards my pill drawer next to the bed and started pounding my Lithium and other psychotropics. As soon as I swallowed, I felt myself begin to calm down, even though I knew there was no way the meds were working yet. Aileen had followed me upstairs and started pressing me as to where I had been, and I told her about the casino. She immediately assumed that I had been with Elle, and requested I bring her to the casino so they could "talk". In my current state of mind, this seemed like a reasonable request.

Aileen was quiet on the entire drive back to the casino. We got inside, passing all the slot machine lifers cranking away, even though it was seven in the morning. I remember thinking how sad that was. But then again, my life was pretty sad, so I probably shouldn't Judge.

I swiped the key card and we walked into the room. Elle was still sleeping peacefully on the bed. Suddenly, Aileen launched herself onto the bed and started pummeling Elle while screeching *"You took my husband to a hotel?!"* Something you should know about Aileen is that she's an absolute pit bull when it comes to physical altercations. She latches on and she does not let up no matter what. There is nothing you can say or do to make her let up for even a second. I would rather fight a grown man than Aileen.

I bolted out the door in a panic, frantically checking the corridor for the police or FBI agents I was sure I heard earlier. I was freaking out, convinced that we were all about to be arrested. I saw nothing in the hallway, so I ran back into the room. Aileen now had Elle by the hair across the room and was slamming her head onto the table over and over, yelling "You will *never* have him! He's *obsessed* with me!" Elle was trying her best to fight her off, but she was like half Aileen's size and, if I had to guess, probably didn't get in fistfights often.

Elle was on the floor now, with Aileen landing blow after blow. I saw blood on the table and started freaking out again. Aileen wouldn't stop screaming, and I knew that people in the neighboring rooms or out in the hallway could hear the fight. I didn't know what to do. I paced back and forth, hyperventilating. Was she trying to kill her? I had to hide from the security cameras!

I went back to the room and the two girls were gone. I hadn't seen them go by me but there was a staircase at the other end of the hall. Evidently, they had gone down to the bar after the fight and got pineapple drinks at the bar. Shit was fucking weird and it didn't stop there.

Elle was pissing blood for the next week trying to heal at home on the couch. Jessica recommended that we terminate Elle and wrote up a legal contract that I never ended up presenting to her. Aileen was fucking lucky that Elle didn't go to the police and press charges like I wish she had done but we had the CPS bullshit going on so she didn't just because of that. It was like Aileen had a license to kill as no one would say anything because of the potential of permanently losing the kids.

136

Lockwood

It wasn't right and of course looking back I wish everything had been different but fear altered everyone's way of thinking and processing, including me.

Every time I told Elle that I wanted to move away with her I was dead serious, however the reality of the situation was very different. Like the drug addict I was, I was not organized and never thought anything completely through. If I were to move away to CT with Elle and Siobhan, I would have to secure housing, work, movers and so forth. Good luck trying to do that with Aileen around.

Aside from that, Aileen had games like manipulation and gas lighting. She would distort my reality to make me question my perceptions, memories, and even my sanity. I began to wonder if the abuse was my fault or that it wasn't abuse at all. I would think things like "I'm the one overreacting, I'm the problem." Yeh, no shit, like the bitch was a fucking magician. She was able to take any situation and make me think I was the cause or the one doing harm. So, you can see that every time I decided to jump ship she had a way to drag me back into her lies and deceit.

The rest of that weekend came and went and Elle came to work that Monday at the office. I couldn't believe it but was ecstatic she was there. Elle was a caliber of person like no one I had ever known before or likely ever will in the future. Even I at the time couldn't appreciate all that she was and would continue to be. That girl saved my life and I can never thank her enough for everything she did and continues to do. I wish I could say at this point that things got better but Aileen had other plans.

Et tu, Brute?

Ian crash-landed at our duplex at around 7:00 p.m. on one of those spring Fridays that feels more like summer. He was Aileen's half-brother, so they shared both a birth mother as well as the traumatic early childhood that she enabled. But unlike Aileen, Ian wasn't adopted young by a rich family. This led to him being very streetwise and much more outwardly troubled. Besides that, the only other thing I knew about him was that he was gay (and preferred Hispanic dudes).

When he showed up on our doorstep, he had just been released from a psych hospital somewhere in Vermont after dealing with some pretty serious psychosis. They basically turned him loose with no follow-up plan. He claimed to be hearing voices but didn't seem to interact with them. I could tell he was in a bad state, claiming that he hadn't slept in days. We quickly ushered him inside and I sprung into action, speaking with him at length to get a full picture of exactly what was going on in his head. I wrote him an antipsychotic that would double as a sleep agent, emphasizing how important it was that he continue to get treatment. At this point, the plan was that he would just crash here for the weekend before returning to Vermont.

Aileen seemed to really like spending time with her brother, and we spent the rest of that Friday night hanging out. Eventually, we started to wind down and we gave Ian one of the unused bedrooms we set up for the kids. Aileen helped him bring a bunch of shit from his beautiful black Acura that he kept immaculate (which Ian had parked on the grass, for some reason) up to the room. After that, he shut the bedroom door for the night, and I was glad the guy was going to finally get some rest. I noticed that Aileen had no issue going into his room even when the door was shut but didn't think much of it at the time. Ian and I did pass each other in the hallway once after that, and he was cordial enough; I assumed that she was probably using their private sibling time to fill his head with lies about how much of an asshole I was ('divide and conquer' might as well have been her motto). Eventually, she joined me in our bedroom. We passed out, and I was grateful for the rare full night of sleep.

Lockwood

I woke up the next day at noon to find the house empty and Ian's car was gone. I took the opportunity to try and look around the room we had given him for the weekend. To my surprise, it was locked. This set my paranoia on edge, so I picked the lock (the doorknobs were the type with a push-button lock on the inside and a hole on the outside, so all I had to do was stick a nail into the hole and the door popped open). Inside the room, my eyes were immediately drawn to the plate of white powder cut into lines. *A fellow cocaine user, awesome!*

I picked up the plate, trying to see if the shit was high-quality. I could instantly tell something was off about the drugs. Most noticeably, the telltale odor of gasoline was missing. This wasn't cocaine, and I wasn't about to taste-test it myself with all the fentanyl going around. I called my friend Scott, a veteran drug addict of all types, and he confirmed my worst fears. Based on my description, he was certain that it was China White, heroin. I was in shock. Aileen's brother does heroin?! Even I had my personal limits when it came to drugs; cocaine was the hardest thing I fucked with regularly. I put the plate back exactly where I found it before leaving the room and locking the door to avoid raising any suspicions.

When they got back, I was down in the basement trying to mount a giant flat screen. Ian offered to help right away, which surprised me. I happily took him up on the offer, and as we worked, I casually asked him what they had been up to that day.

"Oh, we just went to see some of my old friends since I was in the area," he replied. I took that to mean that he was getting established with some dealers in the local area. To be honest, I couldn't blame him for that, but why go through all that trouble if he was just staying for the weekend? I really didn't know what to make of the whole situation, so I started to make a plan in my head. I told Ian that I was trying to have some friends over that night and that he was welcome to join us.

I called Scott again and invited him over that night to help me parse what was going on, as I was completely unfamiliar with the opiate world. He showed up at around 10:00 p.m. with some random chick and a guy who looked like a cop (obviously, Scott didn't fuck with cops, but you know that type of 'look' I'm talking about). The six of us gathered around the dining room table and started socializing. We eventually started trading war stories, with Ian's the most interesting by far. The night was going well; Scott wasn't being too obvious in his observation of Ian, but I could tell he was definitely sizing things up.

After an hour or so, Scott excused himself to step outside, motioning for me to follow. He pulled out a meth pipe and lit up before passing it to me (I usually went pretty easy on that stuff; it'll keep you up for days). In between hits, I asked for Scott's opinion on the Ian situation. Sure, he wasn't doing anything blatantly obvious like nodding out at the table, but Scott confirmed my suspicions: he noticed the remnants of scarred-over track marks on Ian's arms. They were faded enough that I wouldn't have seen them if I wasn't specifically looking, but I could definitely see them when I looked again once back inside. That sealed the deal for me: Aileen's brother was an opiate addict. Obviously, I had a hunch based on the plate in his room, but it made me feel better to have confirmation from an experienced third party.

Saturday turned into Sunday turned into Monday, and it became clear that Ian had no intention of leaving anytime soon. On the bright side, he was actually an excellent cook and I ate better than I had in months. He also kept Aileen occupied and out of my hair, even though I knew that they were probably doing dope together. I was just thankful that I was finally able to have a successful week at work with Elle, staying on time with appointments and therefore minimizing any extra work. Unfortunately, the stability was short-lived.

It started with Aileen deciding that the office would be a fun place to hang out with her brother, and she fell back into her old routine of loudly making videos for social media in the waiting area during business hours. Then, the two of them decided to paint the waiting area, with each wall in a different dark primary color. The place looked like a circus. I was so tweaked out at the time that I didn't question anything about the painting project: the color choices, how it was taking them almost two weeks to paint a couple of walls (it was the perfect excuse for Aileen to spend even more time at the office, 'supervising' my every move), or the fact that they somehow managed to spill an entire gallon of dark blue latex house paint across the carpet of the office waiting room. For days, Elle spent every second of downtime in between calls on her hands and knees, scrubbing the stain with a massive arsenal of carpet cleaners and graffiti-removal chemicals that she purchased with her own money (miraculously, she was eventually able to get the massive stain out of the carpet). I also didn't notice that Elle was hurt and confused by their painting project; my promise that she could design the office had long since left my mind.

Finally, Aileen couldn't drag the project out any longer and the room was just about done. She came to me one night and told me that her brother needed a job. Why not keep it in the family? She suggested that Ian could do the front desk work, and we would get rid of Elle. I brushed her off at first, but she and Ian started to push the matter more and more until it became a problem for me. I agreed to shut them up, originally planning to just let him shadow Elle without actually giving him her position. I figured he would be bored and not want to do it, just like Aileen was.

Monday morning of the next week, I had Elle start training with Ian, while Aileen sat with them to 'supervise'. Elle was immediately uncomfortable and suspicious. That afternoon, she left Aileen and Ian at the front desk under the guise of going to the bathroom and peeked her head into my doorway. "Hey," she whispered. "This has been...weird. I heard Aileen and her brother talking – you're not giving him my job, are you?"

"No!" I faked a laugh. "Oh, God, no. No, you're fine. This is just, you know, in case you have to take a sick day or something." In my mind, I actually thought that this sounded convincing. Looking back, it was obvious that she could see right through the lie. I had been insanely distant to her for weeks but barely noticed; the last time I paid her was almost two months ago, I kept her blocked on my cell phone at all times so Aileen didn't see a message come through and get pissed, and I kept our in-person interactions around the office to an absolute bare minimum as long as the siblings were around (which was all the time, as of late). I had a lot going on in my life between the drugs, Aileen and her brother, and the nosedive my mental health was taking. Adhering to any standards of "communication" or a "healthy relationship" was the furthest thing from my mind, and besides, it's not like she didn't know I was married. In fact, in hindsight, I had really only interacted with Elle twice in the prior two weeks:

1. After being up for three days straight, I became paranoid and vaguely accused her of something, speaking in code, as I left the office. Confused, she told me that it was cold out and offered to get my coat from the closet. I said sure, then

snuck out the door and towards the parking lot as soon as she turned her back to go get it. As I pulled out of the parking lot, I saw her come out of the front door of the building, carrying my coat and looking around like an idiot.

2. One day in the middle of their painting project, Aileen and Ian had to make a Home Depot run to get some more supplies. While they were gone, I called the office phone from my cell. When Elle answered, I asked her to come into my room for a minute. When she got there, I asked her if she wanted to hook up and she said yes. After we were done, she asked me if I was getting any of her messages on Telegram (an encrypted chat app that I had her download after we first hooked up, so we could chat in private). "Oh, I uninstalled that a *while* back. I actually think I hear the phone ringing out there, so I'll talk to you later," I replied (the phone wasn't ringing, but I wanted to make sure she was out of my room and settled back at her desk well before Aileen and her brother returned).

I know how bad all of this sounds, but I cannot emphasize enough how awful things were in my life. Any perceived socialization between Elle and I would result in a guaranteed verbal beatdown courtesy of Aileen, if not worse. I was using meth more frequently and probably sleeping once or twice a week. And I was running into issues accessing my online accounts more often than not, followed by Aileen and Jessica in my ear trying to convince me that Elle was behind it. They repeated it enough that it was an easy thing for my paranoia to grab onto.

The next morning was Tuesday, and I wanted a chance to talk with Elle alone. I unblocked her number and gave her a call when I knew she would be on her way to the office, telling her to meet me at my house instead. "Ok, but I'm literally already pulling into the office parking lot and I see your car here?" She pushed back, but I insisted that I was home. She predictably arrived at the duplex before me to find the door locked with no answer. I told her to go through the backyard and enter the house through the unlocked sliding glass doors to the basement. She texted me back to say that the basement doors were locked. I left Aileen and Ian at the office and drove to the house. When I got there, I could tell she was confused and annoyed by the whole ordeal, especially when I said that there was nothing we needed to do at my house and I just wanted to give her a ride into the office.

On the ride back to the office, she told me about how she got caught on the fence when she climbed over it to enter the backyard as I requested, and everything spilled out of her bag. She was worried that the neighbors would think that she was a criminal, tugging at the locked back door. Then, she proudly pulled out the fancy label maker she purchased to aid in our current project of moving all patient files to an analog pen-and-paper system, due to my recent anxiety and paranoia surrounding online accounts. To purchase the label maker, she borrowed the $60.00 from her dad, on account of her whole "not getting paid" thing. It was the longest conversation we'd had in a while, and I couldn't bring myself to tell her that I was replacing her with Ian.

We arrived at the office with a little while to spare before the first patient of the day. Elle started clearing out the office voicemails from the night before, explaining each step to Ian. The awkwardness between them hung noticeably in the air. Meanwhile, Aileen kept careful watch over the process. She was barely able to contain how giddy she was about the 'secret' - Elle's upcoming firing and subsequent humiliation. I disappeared into my room to prepare for the clinical day.

By mid-morning, Aileen and Ian had to bounce. He wanted to go back to the house, and she had some sudden all-day commitment that required her to drive several hours away (picking up a new set of chicken eggs to incubate from a breeder up in farm country? Something like that). Elle was back at the desk, alone, and could finally work in peace. We had a lot of work ahead of us to "un-digitize" the practice, printing out every intake packet and consent form and getting them into labeled manila folders.

Elle continued this process for the next hour or so, stopping every so often to fight with her new label maker. It was clear she was relieved to finally spend a few hours away from the bitch who openly hated her. She probably even took the siblings' absence from the office as proof that my lie about the safety of employment was actually true. If I were her, I might have even felt a little relaxed, for the first time in a while. Over the noon break hour, she even felt comfortable enough to knock on my door to remind me that she was mostly done submitting my board certification renewal online, she just needed me to fill out the last page with payment information. To her, things probably almost felt normal for a little bit.

Eventually, my first patient of the afternoon arrived. He'd been with me for almost a decade, but I hadn't seen him in person in years. When I grabbed him from the waiting room, he was extremely anxious, almost to the point of panic. I asked him what was going on, and he warned me about "that scrawny bitch at the front desk, walking back and forth, stealing files". As far as I knew, this patient had never lied to me before, so I pulled the security camera app on my phone and watched the live feed of the front desk area. I saw Elle walking back to the front desk with a folder in her hand.

The scene from the camera, along with the patient's increasingly loud insistence that he saw her "walking back and forth" to and from the closet (where the new folders and printer paper were stored), was enough to push my exhausted brain over the edge into delusion. Elle was stealing files from me!?

The rest of the day was a blur of insanity punctuated by the rare lucid moment. I called the police right in the middle of the patient's session before experiencing a brief moment of regret, frantically texting Elle *get the fuck out cops coming NOW* (except with a ton more typos). Then, before she could leave, I ran out into the waiting room and pushed her down, suddenly angry again. With my full body weight keeping her pinned to the ground, I screamed "*If you tell the hackers about this, I'll kill you!*"

"What??" she wailed in confusion. She was crying. "Ok, I'm trying to fucking *leave*! Get OFF." It was chaos. I felt myself yelling but couldn't hear the words. Down the hall, the patient was still ranting. I stood up, and she bolted out the door.

I returned to the session, and soon the cops showed up. I was a little more composed at this point and gave them her contact information. I remembered that they asked very few questions, the first of which was if she had ever done this before. I answered truthfully and told them no. How long we had known each other, etc. And then the obvious: what happened? Well, we saw her walk back and forth from the storage closet to her desk holding a file folder. And what was missing? Nothing that I could see. The situation had calmed down, and the local cops probably already had me pegged as a crazy person, thanks to the multiple vindictive calls Aileen had put in over the course of the last few months. I decided against showing them the "video evidence" of Elle taking a folder from the supply closet and sitting down at her desk with it (mostly because the folder was fucking literally still sitting on her desk).

In the meantime, she had fled the office, and I only heard her side of things later on. Her car was still at my house, so she ended up running to an office park about a quarter of a mile away. The drive from the office to the house was short but unwalkable, including a dangerously busy commercial intersection and a little bit of highway. Her bank account was empty so Uber was out of the question. She had six dollars in her pocket, so she called a taxi service and prayed. The driver was an old Chinese guy who saw how distressed she was and took pity on her, refusing to charge for the drive (she ended up giving him her cash as a tip).

Once back in my driveway, she got in her car as the cops were calling her. They barely had any questions for her, but she offered to meet with them in person (I later found out that this was the first time she had ever had the cops called on her). They welcomed her to meet with them back in the office parking lot, and she agreed. She was so rattled that she clipped my mailbox with her driver's side mirror on her way out, leaving it dangling by a wire.

In the parking lot, she asked the cops if they wanted her to get in their vehicle. They asked if that would make her more comfortable (I think everyone was a little confused by this point). She offered up her purse and car for a voluntary search, and the cops basically laughed it off, letting her know that they were aware that no theft had taken place and she was just doing her job. The only real question they had for her was whether or not I had any problems with mental illness that she was aware of. She actually covered for me and told them no, not that she was aware of, and insisting everything had been professional before today. They reiterated that she was not in any trouble whatsoever, suggesting at most that she would go home for the rest of the day and start looking for opportunities elsewhere if she was feeling unsafe after today.

However, Elle knew me better than that, and came back. When I got in my car to leave the office at the end of the day, she had just pulled into the parking lot. She got out of her car and came over to my window. Before I could say anything, she put her hand up. "Stop. I don't care."

"Are you recording me?" I asked, traces of paranoia still lingering in my mind.

"Fucking what, dude? No. Nobody got in trouble, they knew nothing happened and when they asked me if you were crazy, I said no," she explained. "I don't even care right now. I just know you need to do your board certification thing before the deadline, and I keep reminding you. I also wanted to tell you I got my dad to Venmo me ten dollars, and I went online and bought you these PDFs of these progress note templates that look super easy to fill out so you can finally take care of that kid that keeps threatening to go to the DOH if you don't get him his records."

I was surprised that she came back and was still trying to help after everything that transpired that day. And she was right about everything, the deadline for my board certification renewal, and the vengeful college kid who threatened to report me to the Department of Health if I couldn't produce his records after I refused to arbitrarily write him more scripts. Something didn't smell right about him, it felt like he was hired.

I weighed up the situation in my mind; how many times had Aileen started a fight at home the second I sat down to take care of either of these two things? Enough times for it to look intentional on her part. But I had to go home for the day. After everything went down earlier, I texted Aileen (leaving out the part where nothing was actually stolen and everything was fine), so she was eager for me to come home and give her all the juicy details of Elle's "arrest". But this could also work in my favor...if Aileen thought I was ripshit pissed at Elle for stealing from me, she would never think that we were secretly meeting up if I went back to the office later that night.

"Ok, yeah, you're right," I agreed. "I'm going to come back to the office at like 10:00 p.m. tonight, swing by and park in the back lot of the dentist's office across the street." Elle agreed, and we went our separate ways.

*   *   *

I left my house at 9:00 p.m., leaving enough time in case Aileen held me up on my way out. It ended up being a non-issue, as she was so enthralled by the way I spun the story of the day's events that she never suspected a thing. I told her exactly what she wanted to hear, and she acted like it was Christmas. I arrived at the office, and Elle showed up right on time.

Far from being in my right mind, I forgot at first that the meeting meant something different to each of us. She thought that her exoneration and our meetup to work meant that everything was back to normal, and I was acutely aware of the expectation at home that she was gone for good. She sat down, eager to get to work. "So, where should we start?" she asked.

"Here," I replied, handing her an expandable file folder I had brought from home. She undid the Velcro and peered inside. Suddenly, she recoiled.

"Uh, what the fuck?" she asked, pulling out the envelope's contents. "Is this the only thing here?" It was a pink plaid lingerie skirt. "Dude. I'm not wearing Aileen's...whatever this thing is. C'mon, this shit is important." Frustrated, she stuffed the skirt back in the envelope and passed it back to me. She was so unaware that we might never spend time with each other again, and I didn't dare break her illusion.

She sent me the PDFs that she bought, note templates, and I printed a few out. Her words started to run together, here was a list of the kid's appointment dates, along with any dosage changes, got it. When did I sleep last? I was moving through molasses. Elle kept trying to get my attention, anything to get me to focus. She even started them off, filling out the kid's name and the date of each appointment and cramming them into a manila folder. I was fully out of it. I hunched over the papers at my desk, just to shut her up. I briefly nodded off, then jolted awake to see Elle with her eyes closed on the couch behind me. I couldn't remember why she was here, and I kicked the couch to wake her up.

"Yeah, I really gotta go home. Long day," she said. She glanced at my desk to find that I had made absolutely no progress. "Ok, I'll write you a note with where we left off." She drowsily grabbed a sticky note and wrote *board cert renewal - all done, just enter cc info and SUBMIT* and *college kid progress notes - already dated w med changes* in her small, neat, extremely distinctive handwriting, and stuck it on my desk. I thanked her before offering to drive her to her car across the street.

I surreptitiously grabbed both the sticky note and the manila folder containing the progress notes as we locked up; Aileen was more than intimately familiar with Elle's handwriting and I needed to make sure the office bore no trace of her before the next day. I drove her across the street to the dark lot where her car sat. Unsure of where to hide or dispose of it, I tried to give her the folder to take home.

"Yeah, no offense, but after today, I'd rather not," she explained. I really couldn't argue with that. "Why didn't you just leave it at work? Anyway, I'm dying of exhaustion. So...see you tomorrow, I guess?" she asked tentatively. I can't even remember how I replied, only that it was some flavor of 'yes'. We both drove off.

I don't know what I expected, but she did show up the next morning. Aileen and Ian had been goofing off in the waiting area but immediately became speechless upon seeing her sit down and start working. I was in the absolute epitome of between a rock and a hard place. Before they could confront Elle and her possibly admit that we met up the night before, I came out of my room and into the waiting area. I took an aggressive stance, glared at Elle, and snarled, "*The. Office. Is. Closed.*"

"Uh, yeah. Okay. Sure." she said flatly, picking up her bag and heading towards the door. As the door closed behind her, she turned back to look at me for a split second, enough for me to register the look of utter betrayal in her eyes and the beginning of a tremble on her bottom lip. Aileen was too busy smirking at her brother to notice. I immediately became consumed with the feeling that I fucked up, and wanted to minimize the damage.

I retreated back into my room without a word and dialed Elle's number. Just like always, she picked up. "*Hey,*" I whispered into the phone. "*Meet me at the coworking space.*"

"Got it, I'm on my way." I immediately softened at the relief in her voice. Since Aileen had gotten what she wanted and hated working more than literally anything else, I assumed she would leave Ian to deal with the phones and I could slip out. But she hung around all day, thwarting my plans to escape and meet Elle. Even worse, she knew that all my patients for the day were virtual, so she spent the day even further up my ass than usual. I didn't even get a moment of privacy to follow up with Elle. Eventually, I found out that she waited at the coworking space for me for seven hours, eventually assuming that my phone call was just a mean joke.

*   *   *

Ian operated the front desk like a monkey trying to do algebra, and it interfered with my ability to run the practice so much that I relieved him after two days. Fortunately, a patient let me know that her daughter was looking for work, and I hired her on the spot (it was just one great decision after another, right?). She was young but had some experience working in healthcare. I figured that I had nailed it, and envisioned being able to mold and shape her to do the job just the way Elle did it – which I now know was a truly ridiculous expectation. Her first day was whatever, not terrible, but she was a little bit annoying. When she left for the day, she told me that she planned to arrive even earlier the next day. I firmly assured her that wasn't necessary, but it was clear she didn't get the hint at first. I finally just quit mincing words and told her not to show up before 10:00 a.m.

That night, I was in dire need of as much cocaine as I could acquire to try and numb everything. Aileen was expecting me to be as thrilled as she was that the "problem" was out of our lives, and I needed to play along so she didn't get suspicious. I played the part, kissing and dancing with Aileen for her rude social media video directed at Elle, set to the song "I Think We're Alone Now". She requested I send a message to Elle to reiterate that she was fired and demand she return her key to the office during a time when we wouldn't be there. I obliged, wording the message in the most sterile and professional way possible. I was secretly hoping that Aileen had forgotten about the key and I could use it as an excuse to meet up later, but of course she fucking remembered. Aileen and I watched from home on the security camera app as Elle went to the office, dropped off her keys on my desk, and went into the waiting area to get her nice label maker out of the reception desk drawer. Her movements were large and theatrical, clearly meant to leave no room for confusion as to what she was doing for anyone watching the footage. She spent less than a minute in the office and it was the only time I had ever seen her without her bag and a jacket. I saw the grainy image of the door closing behind her as she left, taking any excuse we had for future contact with her. I never acknowledged ghosting her about the coworking space, and I was eager to do anything to push the guilt out of my mind. She probably hated me by now.

I called my dealer to see if he was around for my usual pickup. He was out of town but gave me his plug's number. The plug answered right away and offered to drive to Bergen to deliver my shit. He ran a much bigger operation, and I got the impression over the phone that he was a bit more polished than what I was used to. He arrived at the office in a blacked-out Jeep, with two girls and his right-hand guy in tow. He was older than I expected but was a nice guy. I invited everyone inside to hang out since it was after 9:00 p.m. at that point and all of the other tenants had long since gone home.

We partied all night, blowing lines nonstop. I ended up hanging IV bags of vitamins for the guests, and everyone was so impressed that they basically thought I was a god. It was a nice ego boost after the shitty week. I soon found out that the two girls were actually hookers who were just spending the evening partying with some drug dealers. Nice girls, just not for me. Eventually, the sun rose over the horizon and by 8:00 a.m. was staring me in the face. The office was a mess, and dread came over me as I remembered that the new girl would be coming in. I decided to be smart about it and reiterate what I told her yesterday, texting her that the power was out at the office and she didn't need to get here until 10:00 a.m. I desperately needed to clean the place up, because it currently looked more like Scarface's mansion than medical practice.

I'll never forget the events that followed. A little before 9:00 a.m., I was standing outside the back door, smoking a cigarette with one of the hookers. I saw the new girl's car pull in, and I instantly knew I was fucked. She saw me before I could sneak inside, and she bounded up the sidewalk towards me with a look on her face like she was expecting me to be impressed that she showed up early anyway, as if she had actually passed some secret "test" by ignoring my explicit instructions. I tried to hide how pissed I was as she flung open the back door and skipped inside.

As most of the previous night's insanity was concentrated towards the back of the office space, she got a full view of the depths of depravity that was my average Monday night. Between the sketchy people passed out with IVs still in their arms and the blatant piles of drugs covering almost every surface, things looked very bad. She audibly gasped in horror before immediately bursting into tears. A few seconds later, she turned to look at me, sobbing *"You're in the same clothes as yesterday!"*

It took me almost two hours to talk her down and get her head straight. I have no idea how I did it or what I said, but I was eventually able to calm her down and convince her in a non-sketchy way to keep what she saw to herself. I played the good guy, and we "mutually" agreed that this position wasn't a good fit for her. With the impression that we were on good terms with each other, she finally left. With that crisis averted, I ushered the rest of the lingering deviants out of my office and cleaned everything up. I must have quadruple-checked every single surface of every single room to make sure that no trace of contraband remained. Somehow, I got everything put back together before the first in-person patient arrived.

With no one manning the front desk, the day was rather bumpy, but I somehow pulled it all off. After I finished with my last patient (conveniently timed to avoid any chance of being asked to work), Aileen finally decided to show up and sit at the front desk, bright-eyed and bushy-tailed after sleeping all last night and all day today. I attempted to work on the day's notes back in my room. Aileen was getting impatient and would storm into my office every time I regained focus. I started to get frustrated and asked for a few minutes of peace to wrap shit up. I had spent every free second in between patients running to the front desk to answer the nonstop phone calls. Voicemails piled up regardless, tomorrow was set up to be even worse, and I couldn't do the job of two people.

Aileen saw a way to leverage my frustration and tried to negotiate with me: she would agree to once again perform her half-ass job of admin for me, until I could find someone new, as long as I paid her. Oh, and she wanted me to send an email to my entire practice, using Elle's full name and telling everyone that she had been arrested for stealing patient files and posing a massive security risk. And she wanted me to include Elle on the distribution list, too. This was just overkill at this point; I had already done the mean thing, I had already done the corporate firing thing, I already knew that nothing was stolen and she had been embarrassed enough. This would be crossing a line, and would no doubt be the nail in the coffin of any chance I had of getting her back.

I protested, using the excuse that admitting such a confidentiality breach would be a terrible look for the practice. But I remembered how not having an admin basically cut my income by 75% when I was virtual; doing it in person would be worse by far. Still, I pushed back, until Aileen's offer turned into a threat. She wordlessly unlocked her phone and showed me her screen, swiping through several photos of me using drugs she had taken without my knowledge. The implication was clear: I send the email, or she would post the photos on social media, send them to my parents and CPS, or possibly even send them to any number of government agencies who could strip me of my credentials.

I begrudgingly composed the email, with Aileen looking over my shoulder requesting tweaks to make it nastier. I knew how wrong it was, but I did as she said. The email was worded as if she was nefariously working under a fake identity and not just using the fake first name I gave her. I exposed her real first and last name, lied that the sheriffs had taken her away after they determined she had stolen confidential patient info, and pinned all computer and phone issues on her. Finally, it was nasty enough to gain Aileen's approval. I made a big show of adding Elle's email address to the bcc field and went out of my way to add other patients' emails as slowly as possible, until Aileen finally got bored and stopped looking over my shoulder. She sighed and told me to just let her know when I was sending it.

The only viable option I saw for damage control was to limit who received it and pray to God Aileen didn't notice. I selected a decent handful of patients, people who either knew the truth about Aileen and would hopefully assume this was nonsense from her, and people who I felt had the highest chance of infrequently checking their email. I finally told her I was sending it off and breathed a sigh of relief when she didn't ask to see the full recipient list.

I clicked the send button and immediately became wracked with guilt. Elle never deserved any of this, and I couldn't believe that things had spiraled out of proportion so terribly. I wanted so badly to contact her in any possible way, just to let her know that I was forced to send the email. But I also knew that it probably wouldn't have made a difference; the earlier shit I could have apologized away, but this was so far into the realm of deranged and unacceptable that I assumed that she would never forgive me.

Over the next few weeks, things got worse in almost every conceivable way. Both my patients and I were reminded of how truly awful Aileen was as an admin. She made it perfectly clear how much she despised the job. The more she whined about not wanting to work, the more my practice seemed to be kneecapped by technical issues (a pure coincidence, I'm sure). Income went down and Aileen's nastiness went up, and she started orchestrating situations where Ian and I would fight (which wasn't difficult, considering we were both short-tempered drug addicts). A fistfight on the staircase ended with me limping for weeks. I became more miserable, did more drugs to cope, and tried my best to ignore the chaos.

A minor bright spot broke through the darkness when I randomly ran into Elle in a strip mall parking lot in Bergen. She waved to me, and I was eternally grateful that Aileen wasn't with Ian and I that day. When she came over to me, I could see how worried she was. I knew how bad I looked; I was still limping, my hair was overgrown, and I had never looked so exhausted. Ian started slinging insults, but she graciously deflected them. I told Ian that everything was cool and asked if we could have a minute.

I wasn't sure if Ian would report the meeting back to Aileen or not, so I knew we had to make it quick. She told me that she had been worried about me this entire time, and I did my best to play it off. I wanted so bad to bring her back, remind her of my true feelings for her, but Ian was nearby. Mostly, I was just so incredibly happy that she didn't want to kill me. We both awkwardly did our best to keep the conversation short and friendly, both acutely aware of the desperate intimacy our energies played out between us. Soon, we could no longer find excuses to drag out the conversation and we went our separate ways. But I finally had hope, and I carried it with me. I didn't want to do that to Elle, she didn't deserve it and by that time I had realized that the whole thing was blown way out of proportion. Elle didn't steal anything; there weren't any files missing. She didn't deserve that. Aileen continued to put pressure on the situation and wanted me to continue to allege accusations that were false.

After another week Aileen had enough as the patient calls and emails had spilled over onto her and Ian and neither wanted to deal with that. Elle was invited back into our dysfunctional universe to admin for my practice. No, people didn't know it was her because it was virtual mostly and I spelled her name wrong on purpose in the email. Besides that, I think most of my patients knew through my squirrely behavior that I was having my own issues. In fact, I know that as people wrote me emails wishing me the best with "whatever it is I'm going through."

A week or so later, I was awoken from a rare night of sleep. It was 3:00 a.m., and Aileen and Ian were going at it again. This was becoming more frequent, and I was sick of it. Our neighbors were even starting to complain. Suddenly, Aileen slammed a door and Ian thundered down the hall and out the front door. He started blasting rap from his car at full volume before returning to the front porch to smoke weed. Frustrated, I leaned out the bedroom window and yelled for him to turn down the music. He ignored me, and Aileen got up in my face, telling me to stop being a pussy and deal with him.

She knew this was a surefire way to get me going, and I soon flew into an adrenaline-filled rage. I grabbed a box of carpenter screws and whipped it out the second-floor window, each one making a plinking sound as it connected with the previously-flawless finish of his Acura. He looked up at the window and started hurling threats and obscenities, amping me up even more. Aileen was in my ear, hissing "*hit him with a bat. Stop being a pussy.*" I was exhausted, hadn't had a rational thought in days, and she kept reminding me that I was being disrespected.

I bolted down both sets of the stairs before emerging from the basement with a broken table leg. Ian was now at the top of the stairs, screaming at Aileen through our bedroom door. I ran up the stairs and swung the table leg at him, hoping to get a good hit or two in while he was distracted by Aileen's bullshit. Instead, he deflected the hit, and we both tumbled down the stairs. I hit my head on the tile at the bottom of the stairs; I was fucked up and had to think of something quick to avoid getting my ass kicked.

For some reason, I decided that faking a seizure would be the best option. I got lucky and the pseudo seizure worked. Instead of continuing the fight, he actually became so worried that he picked me up and led me up the stairs to my bedroom. Out of the corner of my eye, I could see Aileen smiling at the situation she created. Ian was starting to panic, asking her if this happened to me often and trying to figure out how fucked up I was. She clearly didn't give a shit, simply happy that she was able to convince us to hit each other. Ian couldn't figure out why she didn't care if I was okay or not.

Another week passed and, surprise, Aileen and Ian had made up — only to explode again when she hit him with a low blow that sent him over the edge. That was it for Ian. He told me he had enough and was heading downstate to crash with a friend. Before he left, he pulled me aside and took me down into the basement for what he called a "real talk." His tone was serious, devoid of sarcasm or jokes. He said, "Look, she's my sister, but I'm done with her. I've got more respect for you at this point."

Ian started unloading all the secrets he'd been keeping for Aileen. He told me that back when he was living two towns over, Aileen would show up with older guys, fuck them for money right there in his place. She also used to get high on heroin with this friend of hers I'd been treating for free. Then, she fucked this "friend" right in Ian's bathroom. Ian wasn't mincing words. He looked me dead in the eye and said, "She's going to screw you over. Big time. You'll end up arrested...or worse. Jail. She's a man-eater."

I should've listened to that guy. After that, he got in his car and drove away. And just like that, he was gone. I never saw or heard from Ian again.

Death by Hacking

Another thing that started escalating again was the fucking hacking. I was running an independent psychiatric practice that depended on me keeping track of countless usernames and passwords. My memory wasn't what it used to be, so I wrote everything down in a spot I could access easily the next day. Back when COVID hit, the last of my in-person sessions had vanished, and suddenly my entire livelihood was tied to the internet – a real Achilles' heel. It made me vulnerable. Anyone trying to break me down didn't have to lift much of a finger. Whether it was a calculated attack by someone with an agenda or just a bored, sadistic housewife looking for a little chaos, the door was wide open.

Let me set the stage. It's a Tuesday morning, and whether I've just woken up or stayed up all night doesn't really matter. What matters is that my first virtual patient is at 10:00 a.m., and the last one wraps at 4:00 p.m. To function at all – let alone think clearly – I need a heavy dose of Adderall or cocaine, which usually requires at least one call and a meetup. Uppers aren't a nine-to-five gig. Dealers have to be reachable at any hour, even first thing in the morning. I haven't eaten in days, not that I care. Just the drugs, please.

Now it's 9:50 a.m. I need to make myself look somewhat presentable and log into my e-prescribing and telehealth platforms. I open my laptop and check my email first. As usual, there's a ton of junk, but one subject line catches my eye: "Username and password reset notification," sent at 3:32 a.m. It's from my telehealth software. I try to log in. No luck. It's now 9:59 a.m., and I'm locked out. I'll have to call the patient instead, but because I'm slammed with back-to-back sessions, I won't get a chance to contact tech support for a reset. Then I noticed my patient booking software has also been reset. Now I don't even know who I'm supposed to see or when.

This kind of thing happens *all the time*. I called it hacking, and there were plenty of people who might have wanted to screw up my world. At least that's what my paranoid mind believed. That kind of scenario became routine. I was convinced it was either a corporate job or the work of someone tech-savvy (maybe Jose, maybe Nathan, who knows). I spent an absurd amount of time resetting usernames and passwords, troubleshooting websites, and installing Yubikeys on every laptop I owned – basically the closest thing to military-grade cybersecurity I could get my hands on. Eventually, I reached out to a good friend downstate who connected me with the head of the NYC cybercrime division. I remember that call clearly. He said what I was describing sounded like *corporate hacking*, a strategy meant to exhaust someone, steal their time, and chip away at their sanity. He also suspected more than one person was involved, given how constant the interference was.

I started to believe Jason might be behind it. If I were pushed out, his share in the company would grow. They'd done something similar to Vlad, so why not me? The hacking hadn't started until we moved back from California. Before that, everything was fine. Once back on the East Coast, I was within physical reach of others at the company, though I never shared credentials. I became worried that maybe they were using scanning software that could lift saved passwords right from my browser. I had no idea where it came from. But with the drugs and the shady people orbiting my life, I wasn't exactly helping my own case.

For a long time, I was convinced it was Nathan (especially during the stretches when we weren't speaking). But later, after a few sober conversations, I started to doubt that theory. I was so out of my mind at times that I even suspected Elle. Looking back, it was absurd, but when you're sleep-deprived and spun out, nothing makes sense.

Another friend of mine, an international CEO, heard me out one night and echoed what the NYC cyber chief had said: "Sounds like corporate hacking." That stuck with me. Everyone I talked to had their own ideas about who might be behind it. Aileen was quick to point fingers, swearing it was Nathan and Elle and insisting we go to the authorities. So we did. I followed her lead, reporting them based on nothing more than her word. I still remember standing at the front desk of the FBI office as they took down the report and gave us the standard, "Thanks, we'll take it from here." Of course, they never did. The crazed accusations of an ex-stripper weren't exactly compelling evidence. And just like that, the mystery behind the hacking continued, uninterrupted and unsolved.

Adderall and Other False Prophets

Years went by, and my accounts kept getting compromised. I lost count of how many times I had to reset the password for my telehealth software. It was absurd. I'm sure the company started to think I was just doing it to myself (which, given everything, wasn't entirely out of the question). But not like this. I was constantly changing my usernames and passwords, stringing together 30-plus character combinations that even seasoned hackers would struggle to crack. I wrote them all out on a whiteboard in the basement and copied them into a leather-bound journal with a strap and a combination lock. I slept with that thing under my pillow every night and wouldn't let it out of my sight for even a second during the day. It was like guarding nuclear codes.

While the hacking nightmare continued without pause, the rest of my life unraveled at a relentless pace. Nathan and Elle drifted in and out depending on the month, and I was working full-time while Aileen either stayed home or "helped" answer the office phone. With CPS having taken all the kids, she had nothing to do but quietly torment me. I was so deep into the drugs that I couldn't tell what day it was, let alone what was actually happening. I kept multiple laptops, burner phones, whiteboards, and locked cabinets, trying my best to keep things secure. But in the end, only one person had real access. And she was right under my nose the whole time.

Aileen knew all my usernames and passwords (especially during the long stretches of time when I was isolated with her) and she had a knack for getting into anything locked. She slept while I worked, so by the time I was crashing, she was just getting up and wandering around the house, looking for something to do. Nathan, Elle, Jose, and eventually even Jessica all eventually came to believe that Aileen was the one constantly resetting my accounts. She was the only one with full access, and like an idiot, I trusted her.

But why sabotage my practice when the income was funding her lifestyle? Looking back, it makes a little bit more sense: between cash from her dad and any "extracurriculars" she was participating in, she still had money coming in. She didn't care if *I* was broke, and she knew that I would cut anyone out of my life if I thought they were hacking me. So, if I was spending too much time with someone and she wanted them gone, all she had to do was convince me that they were the "hacker" (not a difficult task, given the mental state I was in). For the most part, I was blind to her process. That's what happens when you're deep in addiction and stuck in an abusive relationship – logic collapses. But deep down, I knew at least some of it was her. She even got into my business email and sent out mass patient discharge notices, actually signing her own name to them. Why she wanted credit for that, I'll never understand. None of the patients bought it anyway; they knew I was already drowning in my own chaos.

The hacking problem drove me to the edge. I can't overstate how much it disrupted my life. It drained my time, cost me friendships, and burned through a lot of money. In a paranoid, delusional state, I clung to the so-called "evidence" Aileen laid in front of me. I never imagined that the person undermining everything was the same one who, in my mind, depended on its success. It didn't make sense to me, which is probably why I refused to believe it could be her. To those I falsely accused – people I should've trusted from the start – I'm sorry. I should have listened. But drugs, money, and the illusion of control can sustain a delusion for a while...until it all caves in, and it did.

Later down the road, without Aileen in my life, I've been able to use a single username and password for everything. Since then, there haven't been any issues. Most of my accounts now auto-login with my permission, and with the hacker gone, the constant stream of 3:00 a.m. password reset emails vanished. It became clear later that a major part of what Aileen was doing was deliberate sleep deprivation. After working all day, I'd stay up late trying to regain control of my accounts. And with no sleep, my bipolar symptoms would quickly spiral out of control. Just one night without rest could push me into psychosis. That was the state she wanted me in: vulnerable, confused, and easy to manipulate. And most of the time, it worked.

It wasn't until I was eventually able to stay with Elle for a week and finally slept (like, *really* slept) that I started to feel human again. I saw, maybe for the first time in years, that a different life was possible. But as I've said before, leaving a sociopathic relationship takes timing, and more than a little luck. If you're fortunate, as I was, you'll find good, loving people waiting for you on the other side. Still, the adjustment is brutal. Once you're out of the chaos, your body crashes from constant adrenaline and fear. It's a withdrawal, both physical and mental. Like coming back from war. Panic attacks would hit out of nowhere, wrecking my days.

Looking back, I didn't even see Aileen's tornado of destruction coming. Her darkness crept in so slowly, so subtly, it was almost impossible to recognize what she was doing. It's a cliché, but it fits: like the frog in the pot, slowly boiling without realizing it. I didn't jump until it was too late.

Mind Trapped in a Nightmarish Prison

Panic is one of the most brutal things the mind can endure. It doesn't matter who you are. Everyone hates it, and for good reasons. Panic hijacks the brain, convinces the body that a threat is real, and launches you into full fight-or-flight mode. There's no reasoning with it. It's irrational, but it feels like life or death.

For those new to panic disorder, it's terrifying. For those of us who've battled it for years, it doesn't get any easier. There's no such thing as a convenient time for a panic attack. You're completely at the mercy of the disorder; when it hits, you're down. Incapacitated. For fifteen minutes, maybe more, you're trapped in the most terrifying place imaginable: your own mind, stripped of defenses, wide open to the darkest corners of fear. It's a waking nightmare, and you feel utterly alone in it.

My first run-in with panic attacks started when I was a kid, though I didn't know what to call it at the time. The only cure back then was having my mom or dad nearby. If they weren't around, I was fair game and the panic monster would creep in. As I got older, the episodes faded for a bit, until they came roaring back into my life in my early twenties. I was working as a SICU nurse, carrying a massive load of responsibility. I was great at my job, and I cared deeply about the patients and my coworkers. But one night, right after I had finished mentorship and was officially on my own with two critically ill patients, the pressure boiled over. Stress that had been simmering under the surface decided to punch me right in the gut.

I ran to the nurse's bathroom with what I thought was just stress-induced diarrhea. But while I was in there, it hit me like a freight train. Suddenly, I was having a full-blown panic attack. My body locked up, my mind started spinning, and I was absolutely beside myself in that tiny room. It felt like hours, though it probably lasted just a few minutes. But that was enough. My brain made a brutal association right then: having a bowel movement meant panic. That connection cemented instantly. And just like that, I was fucked. It felt like the worst possible thing that could've happened to me at that moment.

Like anyone else desperate to survive panic, I went on Xanax – and the system didn't hesitate to hand it over (I was a SICU nurse at Yale, after all). It started small: 0.5mg XR as needed. That turned into a daily routine. Then a second dose at night just to get some sleep. Before long, I was up to 1mg XR three times a day, with an extra 0.5mg for "breakthrough" attacks. Even with that pharmaceutical armor, I still unraveled anytime I felt the slightest stomach twinge. I refused to eat, dropping 50 pounds. Completely emaciated, I looked like a ghost of myself. I remember my nurse manager commenting on my weight loss. I was a disaster.

Every shift in the unit became a showdown between me and the panic monster. I tried to outrun the fear, suppress it, smother it with meds, avoid it at all costs. But somehow, it always found me. Eventually, the panic started following me home. It stopped caring about shift hours. My entire life turned to shit; it was consuming me. Panic is brutal like that. The more you fight, the more it wraps itself around you, like a snake, squeezing tighter every time you struggle. That's when avoidance kicks in. Totally irrational, but the conditioning runs so deep that you start reorganizing your entire world around fear. I'd avoid foods I ate the day an episode hit. The color of the scrubs I wore. Specific parking spots in the garage. I realize how insane this must sound, but to me, it was very, very real. You can't avoid everything in life, but I came as close as I possibly could. Somehow, I kept working in the SICU while that thing had me by the throat. Panic had total control over me. Over time, I became aware of the sick irony of it all: the harder I fought, the more it would take from me.

In the decades since, I've learned that the only way to take power back is to stop giving panic that control. If it's going to happen, then I have to let it happen. The longer the stretch between attacks, the lower the chances of having another one. Your sense of self, whatever anchors you, has to be strong, because panic can't survive pure logic and full acceptance. Panic thrives in the shadows of "what if." It feeds on fear, not fact. And the second you start believing thoughts with no credibility, you've already given it an opening.

Still, having panic attacks remains one of the worst experiences imaginable. The one saving grace is that they eventually burn themselves out, leaving your brain so depleted it forces you to rest. I remember feeling completely wrecked after a solid episode, like I'd run a marathon on no sleep. Panic throws the brain into overdrive, with neurons firing like a war zone. That kind of activity isn't sustainable for long.

Biologically, panic was designed to get early humans out of danger fast (think split-second survival reactions, not long-haul suffering). But we're not running from predators anymore, and this ancient reflex has long outlived its usefulness. In today's world, a true panic-worthy moment would be about protecting life, not tearing it apart. I guess what I'm trying to say is that nowadays, panic has become a relic, an outdated response that now mostly haunts the mentally ill (lucky us!).

So, what do you do? That's the big question. One major win I had was during an attack where I literally told it to take a hike. Don't come back unless you've got something rational to say. Otherwise, fuck off. And...*it worked*. The power of that moment was so strong that the panic went dormant for fifteen years. I was so struck by the victory that my brain locked onto it and kept moving forward, panic-free, until everything started to unravel again in my forties. That's when the symptoms began creeping back in. But honestly, wouldn't you panic too if you were staring down seventy months in federal prison? I knew deep down that I could survive it if it came to that, but fear doesn't care about logic. That old feeling of being trapped returned after years of silence, and it hit hard. It's the worst kind of panic I've ever known, like I was drowning and I had no more air left in my lungs. I had to dig deep and hold on to whatever inner strength and logic I could find just to stay afloat.

I believe the key to living with panic disorder lies in finding strength through vulnerability, whether you've had one episode or years of them. It only takes one to understand just how terrifying it can be, and from that moment on, you will do just about anything to avoid another. When I look back on that episode from fifteen years ago, the one where I told the panic to take a hike, I realized it wasn't actually about defeating the condition. It was about accepting what it means to be human. Yes, I'll have bad days. Yes, I will face stress and gut-wrenching physical symptoms. But it's up to me to decide how I interpret that energy. You cannot win by fighting your own primitive survival instincts. Instead, you have to give them space. Recognize them. Acknowledge their presence. And move forward, not as enemies, but as reluctant companions. If and when another episode shows up, take a moment to really examine it. Be honest and objective about how and why it happened. Panic always shows up for a reason, even if that reason is not clear at first (or if it's something you've been trying to ignore).

Panic attacks are primal survival responses, but they can be disarmed if you're willing to work with the energy. They tend to show up when we feel trapped, unheard, powerless, or deep in denial. Over the past year, I've been living with Elle in a calm, grounded environment, and in that space, I've found clarity and peace. Lately, though, I've been dealing with some family issues and noticed emotional volatility creeping in, disrupting my calm. I've even felt the early physical signs of panic – not full-blown episodes, but familiar warnings. It's a reminder that panic disorder can return if I fail to recognize it for what it is: internal energy demanding attention.

When the brain hits a breaking point with stress, panic hits hard. That's usually when someone makes their first appointment with a psychiatrist, desperate to make sure it never happens again. It doesn't matter how they feel about mental health care, panic overrides pride. They're in intense cognitive pain and have no idea how they got there, which is a dangerous mix. I still describe my first episode as feeling like being dropped into a jungle in Vietnam, high on LSD, with bullets flying. That's the level of chaos. So now we have someone like that, blindsided at work, looking for answers. He's booked with someone like me, a psychiatric nurse practitioner. Let's call him Mark.

Mark shows up to my office desperate for answers. He's unsure about therapy or meds. He probably doesn't even realize that he had a panic attack. He only knows that, whatever it was, it cannot happen again. So I get him to tell me a little about his life. He's married to Julie and they have two kids. In the past, Mark identified as bisexual, but never explored it. Deep down, he may align more closely with being gay, though he's not fully aware of it. At work, there's a male colleague he's close with, but on the surface it stays professional. At least consciously. It's a dramatic example, but it gets the point across.

Mark has reached a subconscious breaking point with his feelings for his colleague while also maintaining a family life that's acceptable to those around him. Unless he's willing to explore this inner conflict, the panic attacks will likely continue. He may not need to end his marriage, but his deeper desires need to be acknowledged. If he can talk openly with Julie and she's willing to accept this part of him, they might be able to move forward together. It would take work, and Mark may need prescriptive medications to keep the panic from interfering with his job again.

The fastest way to treat Mark is with a benzodiazepine like Xanax or Klonopin. These meds act quickly by calming the amygdala, the brain's fear center. But most providers won't prescribe them on a first visit (most likely part of the reason why I'm not practicing anymore). While the medication gives Mark immediate relief, it also allows him to avoid facing the deeper issue. Each time panic hits, he silences it without understanding why it's happening. Over time, he needs more of the drug to feel the same effect, until it stops working altogether. Eventually, the panic returns, leaving him right where he started. Most people want a fast solution, but real progress comes from doing the inner work. Finally ready for a real change, Mark starts serious psychotherapy on a weekly basis so he can gain some true insight and take control of his situation. After months of weekly sessions, Mark finally understands what he was feeling, and the panic immediately starts to fade. He's now able to face the situation head-on. His wife's acceptance gives their marriage a chance to grow even stronger.

Often, the thing we're running from is far less threatening than what our minds build it up to be (AC). Logic rarely guides our avoidance, and we pay for it in mental pain. For me, staying grounded and ready to handle problems as they arise is a discipline I have to keep sharp. Clear communication with the outside world helps prevent irrational thinking, but it's easy to lose sight of that. The brain needs open pathways to process thoughts clearly, and substances like alcohol or THC, along with sleep deprivation or chronic stress, can quietly erode those channels.

Panic disorder is a fight worth having as to keep it in check means you are living honestly, rationally and cleanly. Do not let life get ahead of you, always be able to face all sides of a situation, most importantly stay absolutely true to yourself and others around you. You're where you are for a reason; nothing is random. Think about it. Everything in your life – your lifestyle, your relationships, your professional world – exists for a reason. There is no luck, only alignment. Everything is happening as it should, for as long as it needs to.

Adderall and Other False Prophets

If you can sit with that, if you can believe that things unfold with purpose, peace becomes easier to find. I used to resist everything the universe threw my way, thinking I could change reality. But nothing worked for me until I learned to stop running away and finally stand up to what I was dealing with. This is just what I've found to work, both with my patients and dealing with the issue myself. It won't replace being able to work one-on-one with a professional, but I've been grateful for the chance to live a more peaceful existence.

I'll leave you with a few final thoughts before returning to the story. As I've said, I've come to accept my pending prison sentence and know I'll get through it. There are solid reasons behind that conclusion. I'm healthy, I'm happy, I'm active in both my sons' lives, and I'm at peace with the universe. Sure, stress hormones like cortisol or norepinephrine still spike, but I no longer view that energy with fear. Instead, I take it as a sign—something is surfacing that needs attention.

I'm no longer afraid to feel, even when the memories are dark. The past six years have been hard. I was absolutely an asshole at times, but I still had a good heart. I was under the influence and in a relationship marked by domestic abuse. I've come to accept all of it. I no longer hide from myself. I've let go of false idols like money, power, and status. I love, and I am loved. I don't expect anything from the universe anymore.

The old fear of fear, the root of panic attacks, is gone. My interpretation of panic energy is completely different now than it was 20 years ago. When it rises now, I meet it head-on. I challenge it – "Is that all you've got?" – and without fear to feed on, it fades. The brain recognizes the illusion and lets go. Mental illness has no strength against grounded logic and self-acceptance. It thrives in isolation, denial, addiction. And I'm not that person anymore.

Ménage à trois at 40

My 40th birthday was no exception to the madness that defined my life at the time. I spent the morning seeing patients, doing what I loved most, helping people. And honestly, Aileen didn't have anything special planned for me, anyway (her contributions to my birthday had so far amounted to her shooting down my idea for a dinner with friends by saying "Friends? You don't have any *friends*" and an ominous threat in the kitchen that morning. She looked right into my eyes before verbalizing her warning: "*I'm going to get you arrested on your birthday.*" I almost wasn't sure I had heard her correctly).

Elle was back in the office, working for me again. Things were very off-and-on with her; Aileen would push me to fire her, eventually get sick of having to work in her absence, then "allow" me to re-hire her. Elle would always come back, spending hours to undo the mess that Aileen had caused while she was "helping" me. One of these days, I was going to start paying her again.

Things were going well that morning, and I almost wondered if I might get through the day without incident. As if she could read my mind, Aileen showed up to the office, looking for something and about to make it my problem. She needed insurance paperwork for the van, finally up and running after the never-ending electrical problem was fixed. She wanted to start driving for a rideshare again and insisted that I needed to come home to help her find the insurance paperwork that needed to be submitted. I had no idea why my physical presence was needed at home in order to complete this, especially when I still had two patients scheduled for the day.

I couldn't remember if anyone on the schedule for the rest of the day was in-person, so I tried to keep Aileen's drama contained to my room at the back of the office. It was almost two hours before I could talk her down to a level that (I thought) was something resembling "calm". She finally agreed to go home, leaving out the back door of the office. I finally made my way to Elle's desk to get a rundown on who she had to reschedule and exactly how much Aileen had fucked up my clinical day.

Adderall and Other False Prophets

Elle was still catching me up on the day's schedule, and I asked her to follow me out the back door so I could have a cigarette. Aileen reappeared from where she had been secretly hiding for the past fifteen minutes, repeating her threat from earlier to get me arrested and displaying a worryingly aggressive posture.

I immediately spotted Elle's car parked nearby, and I jumped in the driver's seat. Elle dove into the passenger seat and locked the doors. Before I could pull out of the lot, Aileen launched herself an inhuman distance and landed squarely on the car's windshield. I grabbed my cell phone and dialed 911 as Aileen started using her foot to kick the windshield over and over again, all while screaming. First, a small crack appeared. She continued kicking as the crack expanded more and more until the entire windshield was shattered and caved-in, inches from my face. I calmly provided information to the dispatcher until Aileen finally locked eyes with me and figured out what I was doing. She jumped off the windshield and took off across the lot before getting into the van and speeding off.

When the cops arrived, they took statements from both Elle and I. They asked her if she wanted to press charges, and she took me aside for a moment to ask me what I wanted her to do. I sat with the question, pondering for a minute. I thought long and hard before eventually telling Elle that I wanted her to press charges. She returned to the officer and let them know.

Elle's vehicle was in no safe condition to drive, but it was late afternoon by now. We made several calls to her insurance, but they said we couldn't get a rental until the next day. To lighten the mood, I talked about how much fun we'd have going out for my birthday that night. But after an hour or two, I inevitably started to feel guilty about Aileen. I called an Uber, telling Elle that I was just heading out to "pick up something for my birthday".

I thought I had been convincing, but Elle called me out right away. "You're going to get Aileen, aren't you?" I did my best to assure her otherwise and told her I'd be right back.

At home, Aileen was pissed. She'd been arrested and released and was ripshit pissed that Elle wanted to press charges. I tried to convince her that the cops had pushed for it, but she didn't believe it. Aileen made me get Elle on speakerphone and asked her about it, while she was secretly listening. I prayed that Elle would read between the lines, and miraculously, she did. The shocked look on Aileen's face was priceless as Elle corroborated my story, somehow coming up with the exact same situation.

Aileen and I spent the next several hours at home, getting ready for a night out on the town. Elle was trapped at the office with her damaged vehicle, and I got so fed up with her request for status updates that I blocked her number. At around 9:00 p.m., I drove Aileen and I back to the office to grab energy drinks from the minifridge. I was surprised to find Elle still there; I asked her if she wanted a Red Bull and she followed Aileen and I back out to the van.

"Are you at least going to call me an Uber or...?" Elle trailed off. "You said I shouldn't be driving this." I agreed and promptly forgot as soon as Aileen and I pulled out of the office parking lot. We arrived at the parking lot to Jessica's apartment, trying unsuccessfully to get her to go out dancing with us. We decided to just go back home for the night.

The next day was Friday, and I texted Elle to pick me up at the duplex. When she arrived, I was shocked to see that she was still driving around with a caved-in windshield. On the way to the office, she told me that she could pick up the rental her insurance was paying for that afternoon.

Always keeping me confused, Aileen texted me that the three of us should go out that night, to make up for the night before. I hesitantly agreed, and Elle and I grabbed her rental car before heading to my house. I wasn't sure what to expect but was happy to get a few moments of peace wherever I could. Aileen was still getting ready, so I ran inside to grab a quick shower while Elle waited in the car.

Once Aileen and I were dressed to the nines, we went back outside and got inside Elle's rental car. I started driving us to the Electric Co., and Aileen pulled something out of her bag to make the night a little more fun: a chocolate bar, filled with psilocybin mushrooms. Aileen and I did them all the time, but this would be Elle's maiden voyage. She pushed back at first, but I convinced her that it was just hippie shit and it'd be fine.

We pulled into the Electric Co. and it was packed, with a line out the door and spilling into the parking lot. It was a warm night, and the girls were all dressed to turn heads. That's when the mushrooms hit me hard. I stopped the car, convinced there was a turtle in the lot and I didn't want to run it over. There was no turtle, of course (the nearest body of water was miles away) but I swerved around the imaginary creature and found a nearby parking spot on the street. We got in line, and I remember thinking how cool I felt showing up to a club with two girls. It was almost enough to make up for Aileen's deplorable behavior the day before.

We made our way inside and it felt like all eyes were on our little group. Justin met us at the bar and took care of our drinks (just like I said earlier, this guy could make anything and have it taste delicious every time. The girls wouldn't even know what hit them). After catching up with Justin for a couple of minutes, the thumping of the house music one floor up became too enticing and we decided to go upstairs to dance.

The staircase was steep, packed, and full of drunk people. We were tripping and buzzed, with Aileen in heels, and we did our best to make it up the stairs in one piece. On the way, we passed a group of guys who checked us out but didn't say anything. The dance floor was a foggy, pulsing scene of techno and lights. We jumped into the chaos and started dancing, fully in it. The place welcomed everyone – no judgment, just energy. Eager to give Aileen and I enough space to dance as a couple, Elle climbed onto one of the stages and started dancing. Within a minute or two, a girl came up behind her and started grinding. It was hot, no lies there. Yeah, some thoughts ran through my head.

Aileen and I continued to dance on the main floor while I kept an eye on Elle. As she made her way off the stage, that same group of guys from earlier tried to box her in. I saw her face – she wasn't having it – and she pulled away from them. She found a place to stand along the wall about fifteen feet away from us. Aileen noticed and started mocking her to me, saying she couldn't dance or handle herself. Honestly, Elle did just fine. If anyone was dancing like a penguin, it was Aileen.

By 2:00 a.m., the mushrooms were hitting us hard in the best way. I figured it was time to head out—I had more drugs waiting at the house anyway. The night had gone unusually well, and that almost felt unfamiliar. But the drive home was rough. I kept thinking every other car had flashing cop lights on top. I was probably going 45 in a 65, just trying to stay in the lines. Somehow, we made it back to the duplex without incident.

Inside, the trip continued. The mushrooms were still going strong, and so was the energy. One thing about mushrooms: they can turn sexual. Not always, but often enough. Aileen could read me, and started digging through her lingerie drawer. Elle was getting ready to pass out on the living room couch downstairs, and I ran down to her with an idea beginning to take shape in my mind. It wasn't the first time I had floated the idea of a threesome by her, and she agreed to come upstairs (probably a combination of the mushrooms, an idealistic belief that she could somehow use her actions during the encounter to convince Aileen to hate her less, and her genuine desire for me to have a good birthday).

Upstairs, Aileen was fully naked under a red mesh tube dress. She offered Elle a baggy T-shirt and a pair of leggings. The three of us settled onto the master bed and watched music videos on my phone until I could feel the tension shift. Both girls looked great, and it didn't take long for my dirtball brain to start racing again.

I had never been in a situation like that and had no idea what to expect, especially considering how volatile things were between Elle and Aileen. We had been hanging out for about 40 minutes, unsure who should make the first move. Finally, Elle, wanting to give me a birthday to remember, turned to Aileen and asked, "Do you want to make out?" Aileen agreed, and she stretched out on her back with Elle's lips pressing against hers. I sat there, stunned, unsure what to do or how to even process what was unfolding in front of me. Both the girls were clearly enjoying it. I was watching something I never imagined would actually happen. Was I really part of this? Was this considered a threesome?

Suddenly, the mushrooms betrayed me.

In an instant, my excitement morphed into confusion. I felt like I needed to protect Aileen from Elle. I rubbed Aileen's head and snapped at Elle, accusing her of trying to steal my wife. The moment unraveled as fast as it had come together. What could've been something rare and unforgettable turned into me yelling, unraveling the whole scene. Aileen probably enjoyed the chaos, but even she was confused.

Elle jumped off the bed as I kept yelling, telling her to go home. She was stuttering, explaining that she was still under the influence of mushrooms and alcohol and couldn't drive safely. I wasn't hearing it, even as Aileen emotionlessly offered "she's probably right" from her spot on the bed. I continued yelling, eventually telling Elle that she could stay here for one more hour, tops. But she had to spend that time on the phone with the police department, doing whatever she needed to do to un-press charges on Aileen for the windshield. She agreed and bolted downstairs.

And that's how I fucked up my shot at threesome.

*   *   *

I did this over and over, and looking back, I see it as an extension of Aileen's anger. Her hatred for the world bled out through me. I became her puppet, lashing out at others when I couldn't carry the weight of it anymore. In this case, I convinced myself that Elle was trying to steal Aileen from me, which wasn't true at all. Delusions like that were common. I projected an unbearable amount of pain onto the people closest to me. Sometimes it came out as irritability, other times as actual harm. There were no filters, no guardrails – just raw pain running the show. I had stopped caring what anyone thought of me; I considered myself nothing more than a waste. And no amount of drugs could numb me from Aileen's darkness. It showed up every time.

This is what's left in the wake of a true sociopath—manipulation, destruction, and chaos. Aileen breathes pain like air. It doesn't faze her. She runs toward it because it's her native language. She used my vulnerabilities against me, shaping my behavior through constant pressure. After six years of that conditioning, she could get me to do things I never thought I'd be capable of, including hurting people. I can think of four separate instances where someone got physically hurt, and each time, she was there behind me, whispering in my ear, fueling it. She even got off on it when I disciplined the kids. I'll never forget the day in California when she pulled me into a room and told me to yell at them for something small. I remember the smile on her face as I got worked up over nothing.

Her operating system is pain, and like anyone exposed to it long enough, I learned how to adapt. It took years, but eventually she had full control – manipulating my behavior until it aligned with her desires. People like Abbie and

Elle saw what was really happening. They knew I wasn't a bad person, just someone caught in a deeply abusive relationship. Most people never escape that cycle. I like to think of myself as intelligent, but it still took a full year of sobriety and stability before I had the courage to leave. In hindsight, I can't believe I didn't do it sooner. That's what the drugs were for, I guess: to help me stay numb and blind to what was right in front of me.

If you're a guy and you're reading this, I bet I know what you're thinking. You'd never blow such a golden opportunity, no matter what drugs or mental illness or abusive dynamics were at play. And before I lived through it, I would have absolutely agreed with you! But I cannot overstate how completely being in a relationship with a sociopath hijacks everything you thought you knew about yourself.

Above all, I didn't want to admit to myself that I had failed another marriage. I completely blamed myself, and Aileen was well aware. She reminded me often, using guilt to pour salt in the still-open wounds I bore from what I did to Abbie. I'd think, how the hell did I mess up a marriage to a stripper? That should've been an easy win. I expected more from myself; I just needed to try harder with Aileen. I needed to show her just a little more care, offer a few kind words, a reminder that I loved her. But none of that would've made a difference. That's not how she operates. Her currency is chaos and pain. Destruction is the only game she knows. Like Ted Bundy once said about murder, "Every time it happened, I thought it would be the last. Like it would fulfill the desire." That's Aileen. She consumes or destroys, then moves on. She wrecked her first husband, and she did everything she could to wreck me too. "She's the reincarnation of Satan," her ex-mother-in-law once said. I didn't believe her at first, but now I know she was right.

Let's be clear about what Aileen is: a calculating predator. In the beginning, she came at me with nonstop praise and affection. It felt incredible, like she actually understood me. I got hooked fast. But almost without noticing, the compliments shifted into subtle jabs. I was "too sensitive," "too dramatic." And when I pushed back, she'd tell me I was imagining it. Over time, I stopped trusting my own memory and started trusting hers instead. I wasn't sleeping, I was on a ton of drugs, maybe I really *had* misremembered things. For a while, there was always just enough plausible deniability for me to ignore the nagging suspicions at the back of my mind.

Suddenly, I was stuck on an emotional roller coaster. One minute she was sweet and affectionate, the next she was cold and distant. When the kindness came back, it felt rare and precious, so I clung tighter. Slowly, she isolated me from friends and family until I felt like no one else understood me. I started to depend on her completely. Then came the fear. She'd threaten what might happen if I left. I had too much to lose. She hinted that her ex-husband was still in the picture, which made me jealous and desperate to keep her close. She talked badly about me to others, even my parents, trying to dismantle every aspect of my support system. When I'd crash from pure exhaustion, she would vanish for hours. That silence wrecked me. It felt like a panic attack every minute I didn't hear from her.

Eventually, I developed a trauma bond. My brain started to confuse love with pain, making it feel impossible to leave. Abuse followed by sudden affection kept me hooked, like my nervous system couldn't tell the difference anymore. The intermittent reinforcement was addictive. I felt loyal to her, even protective, like I owed her something. That cycle of hurt, then comfort, then hurt, trapped me deeper than I ever imagined. All the while, we were becoming further linked in the traditional sense (a shared child, marriage, etc.). Extricating myself from her felt impossible, especially when she always made sure I had a more-immediate crisis monopolizing all my attention.

Now you can see why people like her are the most dangerous ones in the room. You don't realize it until it's too late – just like I didn't on February 21, 2017, the night we met. I was desperate and broken, and she saw it all. She knew exactly what she was doing, and I walked straight into her trap without even knowing it.

Lockwood
On the Edge of Salvation

It was the brutal end of June, with temperatures stuck in the high 80s: perfect conditions for short tempers and impulsive decisions. I was still trying to process the chaos of the past few weeks. Aileen's father threw enough money at the management company that they let us break the lease for the office early, so I once again returned to working virtually. Jessica accompanied Aileen to her court date for Elle's windshield, and Aileen got off scot-free, as usual. The circumstances surrounding this were less-than-ideal; Jessica wrote up paperwork saying that Elle's windshield had actually been caved in for a while and she wasn't sure how but it *definitely wasn't Aileen,* no way no how. Elle agreed to sign it when Jessica insisted that I'd have no shot of seeing Lorenzo again if she didn't. As soon as the signature was obtained, Aileen orchestrated a situation where she was able to convince my sleep-deprived ass to physically shove Elle to the ground in my driveway before calling the cops on her.

I spent the next week or so wracked with guilt until I could re-establish contact with Elle. Forgiving as always, she agreed to meet up with me at the new coworking space where I was trying to work. Things felt safe enough, all things considered, and I asked her to work for me again. Aileen spent the next few days emailing me threats, posting naked pictures she'd secretly taken of me online, and discharging my practice via email again. I had another tearful phone call with my parents, this time I asked Elle to move to Connecticut with me, and convinced her to leave her car in a parking lot overnight (it got towed). Once Aileen turned on the sweetness, I for some reason ran home, leaving Elle alone in the parking lot of a CVS with empty promises to return in 30 minutes.

And that's where I found myself now, at home, with only Aileen and my own bad decisions to keep me company. Things were miserable. The sliding basement door was still broken, letting all the cool air escape. Down there, it reeked of chicken shit and buzzed with flies. I had finally given up trying to manage her birds. Every time I made progress, they'd take back more space than before (sound familiar?). She knew I didn't want them there, but at that point, I was too worn

175

down to care. I was out of drugs, out of money, and for once, trying to focus on myself – no one else, not even her.

Without money to put gas in the car or minutes on my phone, Aileen had me locked in a perfect storm. I was completely at her mercy, and she loved every second of it. Watching me squirm gave her a kind of thrill, knowing that the lack of control was eating me alive. To make matters worse, my online patient booking system was down (Aileen's doing, without a doubt), so no one could schedule appointments. I was stuck, cornered, out of options. I checked the van: less than half a tank. Maybe enough to escape.

I managed to get one call out to my father in Connecticut (I had pretended to be asleep and Aileen left her phone unlocked when she went to take a shower), telling him what was happening and letting him know that I was going to try and make it to their house on the fuel I had. I had no choice. She had plenty of money from her father but kept it all from me. I knew if I didn't leave right then, I risked being completely paralyzed.

The trip to Connecticut was just over two hours, and like my father and I had discussed, taking the back way down Route 8 gave me a better shot at making it before the tank reached E. "Go fuck yourself, Aileen, honestly," I muttered to myself as I peeled out of the dirt driveway that Thursday morning. I left the house with nothing but my meds and the last shred of optimism I had. It was a beautiful day, and if I drove carefully, I knew I could stretch what fuel I had. I didn't know exactly what I'd do when I got to Saddlebrooke, but I knew I had to get out from under her. I was a slave in that house.

The van's CD player had one album in it, *Westside Connection*, and I played it on loop. I got off the highway in Lee, Massachusetts, and started the rural stretch of Route 8. When I say rural, I mean West Virginia rural. If I broke down out there, I wasn't sure who – or what – might find me. The fuel gauge was dropping faster than I liked, so I stopped at a tiny mom-and-pop gas station, one of those old-school joints where a bell rings when you pull in. I had exactly $4.97 in change in the console, just enough for a little over a gallon and a half. About 25 more miles of range.

Lockwood

An older guy came out to pump the gas, with a piece of hay in his mouth like something out of a movie. He clearly knew I wasn't local, clocking my desperation right away. Still, he didn't ask questions. We made small talk, and he ended up topping me off with $6.00 worth but only charged me what I had. I was struck by his kindness. As I pulled away, I thought there are still good people in the world. Aileen was not one of them.

I made it to I-84 with about 20 minutes left and barely an eighth of a tank. I held my breath as I burned through the last sliver on the gas gauge (thank God that old man topped it off), exhaling only when I knew I was safe in Saddlebrooke at last. I met my father, who filled my tank, bought groceries, and set me up in my brother's unused condo. He even handed me $50.00 for spending money. He could see I was wrecked and left me alone to rest.

That night I sat in silence, staring at the walls of the condo, trying to make sense of what my life had become. I desperately tried to imagine a way forward but kept hitting dead ends; my brain was completely steeped in hopelessness. I felt completely trapped no matter which way I looked at it. I had been in over my head for years and there was no conceivable outcome that led to peace or happiness for me. With no way out, I decided I could at least put an end to my suffering. I took 25 milligrams of Klonopin and chased it with half a bottle of Ketel One I bought with the money my father had given me. I remember the warm wave that washed over me as I laid back, hoping my breathing would just stop. The pain finally lifted, and I welcomed the feeling. At that moment, nothing mattered – not even my kids. That's the brutal truth, and it's hard to admit.

Looking back, I can't believe I had allowed someone to reduce my life to that point. She didn't care what happened to me, or how her torture made me feel. By now, she was intimately familiar with my pattern of behavior and knew I'd be trying to escape. I'd begged her for gas money the week before and she refused. She had thousands of dollars from her father stashed away and didn't offer me a dime. She watched me struggle and did nothing. But I didn't want to give her the satisfaction of being my final earthly thought, and I let the pleasant numbness wash over me.

Adderall and Other False Prophets

*   *   *

Bang, bang, bang. "Asher, please open the door." It was my father. Time: 1:00 p.m., Friday. I hadn't died in my sleep. I was awake, aware, and pissed off. I couldn't even kill myself properly. I knew the math. I knew what an overdose looked like with that drug. Maybe my decade-plus on Xanax had built up enough tolerance to fuck that up, too.

I opened the door. He looked at me and said, "You look like death warmed over, Asher. What did you do last night?" He didn't realize how close he was to the truth. I brushed him off. He had errands to run and asked if I wanted to come. I said yes, which was my first mistake. After that much Klonopin, your mind isn't right (no matter how cool, calm, and collected you seem). I played it off, but internally, I was still numb.

As we drove, I noticed he was heading towards his home. The problem was, CPS had told me I wasn't allowed to see Lorenzo, and that's where Lorenzo was. I told him I couldn't go there. He sped up. My mind spiraled – was he setting me up? Was CPS going to be there? The cops? What the hell was happening?

The closer we got to the family home, the more panicked I became. We reached a four-way stop and my father tried to roll through it. I didn't care. I opened the door and jumped out, the car still travelling at ten or 15 miles per hour. Whatever. I was done. He kept driving toward his house and I stood there, at the intersection, trying to catch my breath. Maybe Aileen was right; I really *couldn't* trust anyone but her.

I was suddenly jolted out of my thoughts as three police cruisers came flying in out of nowhere, lights flashing. "Get on the ground! Hands where I can see them!" I couldn't believe it. What the hell was this for? I couldn't believe my own family had betrayed me like this.

They cuffed me and sat me on the curb. That's when I got a good look at them – young guys, all of them. I actually recognized a few from the town's summer swim club growing up. Then more cops pulled in, and I just kept my mouth shut. I knew better, especially in the state I was in. Moments later, an ambulance rolled in quietly, with no lights or sirens. Just like that, I was the center of a scene I didn't even see coming.

Car after car drove by, each one seemingly driven by someone I recognized. It was humiliating. One of the officers finally told me I needed medical care and that the EMTs would take over. I said no. I just wanted to leave on my own. Then the chief stepped out from the shadows and said, "You need medical attention. Please get in the ambulance." I agreed, mostly to get away from them and avoid any further issues. I've never been a huge fan of cops. Some are good people, but others abuse their position.

Inside the ambulance, it was just one EMT and a driver. It seemed understaffed, but I went with it. Better than sitting in a holding cell all night. I laid back on the gurney while we started moving. About halfway into the ride, my back went into a full spasm – possibly a withdrawal effect of the massive amount of Klonopin I had taken. The pain was unbearable, like my entire spine was locked in a vice. I told the EMT what was happening, but he didn't respond. I couldn't figure out if he didn't hear me or if he just didn't care. Looking back, I think he was waiting for an excuse to escalate things.

Eventually, I stood up, desperate and in pain. He immediately flinched and said, "Please don't hit me." I wasn't anywhere near him, and I wasn't even holding up a fist.

"I'm in terrible pain," I said, as calmly and clearly as I could. That seemed to be the opportunity he was waiting for. A moment later, he injected me with Versed and put me out.

It was two full days before I woke up in the same hospital where I was born. I probably needed the sleep. Nurses and residents were buzzing around, and I noticed my flow sheet on the bedside, that 24-hour documentation of everything. I felt calm, clear, and starving. What the EMT didn't realize was that I had already taken 25 mg of Klonopin the night before, and the 2 mg of Versed he gave me only compounded the effects. It acted like a moderate sedative, which makes sense since Versed and Klonopin are basically first cousins. Lucky me.

Adderall and Other False Prophets

A nurse came over and I asked all the usual questions – where was I, what I was being held for, etc. Since I had been labeled "combative" in the ambulance, they kept me in the ER for observation to make sure I wasn't still a danger to myself or anyone else. That's psych's job in a setting like this: assess safety first. And, oddly enough, I *did* feel safe there. The staff seemed to genuinely care, and I missed being around other medical professionals. When a tray of food finally came, I ate every bite, even the condiments. Then I crashed again, drifting back to sleep as the staff kept an eye on me.

In the meantime, word had gotten out back in New York that I'd been taken to a hospital. Both Aileen and Jessica started panicking. If I got admitted, Jessica would lose her Adderall supplier. They began pinging my parents with questions, but, unbeknownst to me, my folks already had a plan in motion. I was set to be transferred directly from the hospital to a six-month rehab program in Kentucky, something I desperately needed at the time. They were just waiting on transport: my parents had arranged for a chartered jet with a personal escort to get me directly to Lexington (a very smart move on their part).

However, my parents failed to understand and account for exactly how strong of a personal motivator addiction is. Even someone like Jessica, who had a professional license on the line, was willing to risk everything and then some, just to keep her line of supply open. As for Aileen? She didn't care about the drugs; she just didn't want me to get better.

Sitting in that hospital bed, I started to clear up mentally and began wondering what the plan was for my treatment. I had been in the ER for days, which was unusual for any patient. Looking back, I wish I had known and understood what my parents were trying to do for me. I needed that help more than anything. Before long, I decided to take a nap to pass some time.

I was mid-dream when I heard a familiar voice, distant and disembodied, saying, "Asher, wake up, we're here." I didn't want to leave the peace of that dream, but I opened my eyes to see Aileen and Jessica standing on either side of my bed. They told me the "good news" – that my parents had tried to force me into inpatient treatment, but they were able to pull some strings to secure my discharge and they were here to take me home. I was relieved to see them. By that point, I was getting sick of the hospital and I just wanted out.

I asked how that was even possible, since I'd been admitted against my will for what they claimed was "aggressive, violent posturing." That's when Jessica chimed in and said she'd told the hospital she was my power of attorney and that my wife was there to pick me up. It was a total lie, I never named Jessica as my power of attorney. But even though the staff knew what the real plan was, they had no choice but to release me. The paperwork looked clean enough to get them off the hook.

My parents had no idea this was happening. By the time they found out, I was already back in New York standing on Jessica's back porch in the sunshine like nothing had happened. My phone rang. It was my mother. I picked up, still unaware of everything that had just been undone. She asked to speak to Aileen and told her, "You're a real piece of shit, Aileen." Then she turned her attention to Jessica: "Aren't you an officer of the court? What you did was illegal, and we have proof."

Jessica didn't have much to say except, "Sorry for the confusion, we were only trying to help." But she knew that was complete bullshit. I took back the phone and hung up the call. I thought I had just dodged a bullet. In reality, it was the first real shot someone had taken at saving my life. I guess it just wasn't my time yet.

The girls explained to me exactly how they were able to pull everything off. All Aileen knew was that I had gone to Connecticut and ended up in the hospital. Jessica told her to call Hartford Healthcare, since they owned all the hospitals and had a centralized database. Because she was listed as my wife, she was told exactly where I was. Once they arrived at the hospital, Jessica did most of the talking. The staff, maybe a bit too casually, revealed that I was being prepped for a private transfer to a rehab facility in Kentucky. Once they had that information, they did everything they could to derail it, and they succeeded. Just like that, I was pulled straight back into the nightmare. And the worst part is, I went along with it. I was the maestro of my own demise, conducting the orchestra as the stage gave way.

My parents tried everything to get me into treatment. They crossed lines, took risks, and made real sacrifices. And all I did was spit in their face. Maybe I wasn't ready for a six-month program – maybe I would've bounced anyway and wasted their time and money. I like to think I would've made it work (maybe it would have even changed the course of the years that followed), but that's lost to time now.

Ultimately, I wasn't ready to fully see the truth yet. I was blind. To Aileen, I was a toy to manipulate and break. To Jessica, I was just a reliable Adderall pipeline. Neither of them is capable of genuine love or human connection. They move through life empty, chasing one hollow dopamine hit after another, never finding peace. "May you live forever," as King Leonidas said, and I mean that for both of them. May they live long enough to see everyone age and die as they walk the earth alone. I don't think either of them will ever be truly happy.

This was no way to live. But I'm one of those people who believes nothing happens by chance. In June of 2022, I was deeper into drug use than ever before, down to 130 pounds from 205. My brain was shot. Planning and rational thought had long since vanished. But I still had access and didn't plan on stopping yet, not while my body was still "healthy" and I felt like I could afford the lifestyle.

Sad, isn't it? I measured how long I could maintain the high, knowing eventually I'd have to quit, one way or another. But for the moment, my family had Lorenzo, Abbie had Giovanni, and I had the capacity for good income along with a soulless companion to share the void with every day. Why stop? The numbness was too convenient. As long as I stayed high, I didn't have to feel or think too much

It felt like it could go on forever, but of course, it didn't. Emotion always breaks through eventually. Vulnerability and guilt were the cracks in my armor, and there weren't enough drugs in the world to keep them patched forever. And what kind of father had I become in the meantime? I was a ghost, sending Amazon gifts to Giovanni for birthdays, hoping that counted as parenting. Abbie accepted them kindly, though I didn't deserve it. But what did my son really know of me? Who was this man named Asher who drifted in and out of his life like smoke?

I can see his face and hear his words even now – "Asher, why did you leave me and Mom?" I brought up that exact interaction at an AA meeting once, and the room went silent. That never happens. Someday I'll have to tell him the truth: that I was afraid of failing as a father, so I ran. I used drugs, surrounded myself with the wrong people, and lost everything. But how can a child understand that? My biggest fear is that he'll think he wasn't enough for me to stay. That he'll believe he (or his mother) wasn't worth fighting for. It'll be a painful conversation; one I'll have to have with both of my sons. But I believe, in time, it might bring us closer. Vulnerability, when embraced, can be a strength. It's the cornerstone of real connection, especially in families.

I know what *doesn't* work in a family: everyone white knuckling their own way through life, never asking for help, ruling through fear. That was the house I grew up in. Life's hard enough with good guidance, and nearly impossible without it. It's okay to be emotionally present. It's okay to feel. I knew that kind of love with Abbie and her family, and, even though it took some time, I eventually found it again with Elle. But I had to stop running – from pain, responsibility, vulnerability, and especially from myself.

I'll go back to what I said earlier: *everything happens for a reason*. I had gotten so used to the painful reality of my life with Aileen that it felt normal by that point. Things would have to get much worse before I was ready to make a change.

Psychosis: Falling Away From Me

Psychosis comes in many forms, but the source is always the same. When the brain is put under extreme stress, it produces symptoms appropriate to the triggering situation. Here's an example: imagine you're sitting in class, and the teacher springs a surprise test on everyone. You know you're completely unprepared, so your brain produces anxiety. You take the test, and it turns out you failed. You know your parents are going to be absolutely livid, and you were already on thin ice at home before this. In response, your brain produces panic. Now imagine that you're abusing drugs like Adderall and cocaine and running on a dangerously small amount of sleep: you start to believe that your teachers are all colluding to spring unannounced tests on you so that you get in trouble at home and can't get into college. Finally, imagine that in addition to everything else I just mentioned, you're also under the constant unrelenting stress of a domestically abusive relationship and are under investigation by the DOH and DEA. The paranoia progresses into a full delusional state where you're convinced that the FBI is watching you from across the road and you can't stand in front of any windows. Your brain is now confabulating reality because it cannot deal with the stress of what is actually going on and you end up in full-blown psychosis. The brain is a sensitive organ that if stressed will do whatever it has to do to protect itself. If that means confabulating reality then so be it.

I may have combined two separate examples in the previous paragraph, but the point still stands: psychosis usually starts as something based in reality but grows and changes into something completely false when factors like stress, drug abuse, and lack of sleep are applied. It even happens in situations like war when a soldier watches a friend's head get blown off. They cannot accept the stressor for what it is, and, in response, confabulate or dissociate from reality which makes things tolerable at best.

During the Summer of 2022, both my abuse of drugs and Aileen's abuse of me increased to new heights. As a result of this, my brain had become very soft and I was easily convinced of various situations and scenarios despite either the lack of proof (or extensive proof to the contrary). Aileen saw my fragile mental state as an opportunity to benefit herself and the empty threats, abuse, and taking advantage of me got even worse than prior. I had so much stress piled on top of me that the lines of reality began to blur. I started to believe that the people who lived in the other half of the duplex were DEA and listening to us through the walls. I also believed that someone was taking the mail out of our box every day (I actually wasn't totally wrong about this; Aileen was hiding important mail from me like letters from the Department of Health and any new debit card I ordered).

Truthfully, I wasn't completely unaware of the fact that she was the one fucking me over, I just didn't know (or didn't want to believe) how bad things really were. Every so often I would stumble onto concrete evidence (ranging from bank statements showing that she had stolen money from me to official notices from the government requiring my response that she wouldn't think to give me until the due date had passed, postmarked weeks earlier), but she was always ready with an excuse or more misdirection. She was adept at using my own paranoia against me and convincing me that it was actually Elle, or Nathan, or the telehealth company I had founded causing all the chaos in my life. However, that summer, she grew bored with the usual threats, violence, and personal and professional sabotage and began employing a new tactic: orchestrating traumatic situations designed to send me into psychosis.

The first serious psychotic episode began during a trip to pick up her three kids for a CPS-approved day visit. She knew her ex-husband would be there and there was a chance that we would run into him, which would have been a tense situation (I knew she had cheated on me before). We were on the highway approaching the exit to pick up the kids when Aileen looked at me and said, "Asher, I didn't want to tell you this, but there are state troopers up here waiting to arrest you." I was immediately overcome with panic and truly believed I saw red and blue lights up ahead. I pulled the van over on the side of the highway and jumped out, running into the woods in sandals, shorts, and a t-shirt. As I cut through the brush, I looked back to see Aileen driving away.

I began to zig-zag my tracks, thinking the police would have dogs to track me. I ran and ran until I got up the side of the hill and found myself on some sort of dirt road. On one side of the road, I saw a graveyard. On the other side of the road was an endless field of cornstalks, with trees in the distance with what appeared to be hunting stands. I suddenly remembered that I still had my cell phone on me, and realized that the police could be using it to track me. I threw my phone into the graveyard without any concern that I would possibly need a way to communicate or get a ride home. The only thing on my mind was avoiding arrest.

Suddenly, I heard gunfire ring out in the distance. I ran into the cornfield to hide so any hunters in the area didn't see me and mistake me for a deer. Maybe that wasn't a gunshot I heard. Maybe there wasn't even a sound at all. It was one of the hottest days of the summer and I had just run for what felt like miles with the July sun beating directly on me with no food or water. Pure fear and adrenaline coursed through me. I found a hiding spot in the miles of rows of identical corn and sat down, deciding that moving around too much might make noise and alert the cops to my location.

Hours passed. I was now completely dehydrated, lying amongst endless rows of corn under the hot sun. When I finally opened my eyes, I could swear I saw men's boots. They weren't right next to me, but close enough that I could see them from my hiding spot on the ground. As I lay sunburned in the dirt, I could feel ants crawling across my arms and legs and biting me. It really hurt, but I didn't move. I started to hear what sounded like men laughing at me, but I couldn't pick my head up in that blazing sun. I felt completely paralyzed, and after a few minutes I passed out face-down again.

When I awoke for the second time, the sun was no longer directly overhead and I guessed it to be late afternoon. I was able to slowly get myself up and decided to continue my trek in hopes of finding an actual town. I had no idea how long I had been running earlier so I didn't know where I was or if I had successfully outrun the police who were looking for me. I kept walking until I reached the other end of the cornfield and houses began to come into view. I passed houses with pools and sprinklers but was too paranoid to knock on a door to ask for water. I was surrounded by salvation yet imprisoned by my mind. I didn't realize it yet, but I hadn't made it too far from the highway exit: I was in the town where Aileen's ex-husband and his parents lived, and they basically ran that place in all but official titles.

Lockwood

I made my way through the neighborhood before finally hitting the main road. I made a beeline for the first gas station I saw and bought a bottle of water with the few crumpled dollars I had in my pocket. I pounded the entire bottle and felt like I wasn't going to die for the first time in hours. The cashier gave me a funny look. I was an absolute mess: I had no car or cell phone and every inch of me was covered in sunburn, ant bites, and cuts from running through brush and thorny bushes.

I left the gas station and saw that dusk was beginning to fall. At this point, I was no longer delusional and hallucinating but still paranoid. It seemed like the locals were staring at me as they drove past, which increased the paranoia. Across the street was a Taco Bell with some people gathered in the parking lot. It seemed like more and more people were joining the crowd, and I became convinced that they were all people I knew who didn't like me. Danger seemed to be everywhere, but I was stranded and needed help.

I scanned up and down the street, looking for any source of assistance or safety. I saw a local police station right by the highway entrance up ahead. I made my way up the street and stood in front of the door to the station. After spending all day trying to hide from the cops, I was now at their mercy. I was in desperate need of help and immediate medical attention and, without a phone or any more money, had no other options.

My plan was to wait for a police officer to drive into the parking lot and ask them for help. In the meantime, my mind ran wild with paranoid thoughts. Strangely enough, I looked back at the gas station to see several state troopers filling up their tanks. I anxiously watched them pull out of the gas station and drive towards me. *How the hell did they know I was here?* I thought, until I realized they were driving right past me, slowly but without interest. *Maybe that's the gas station where they usually fill their tanks?* One of them pulled up to the pump, got out and stood in front of it but decided to get back in her cruiser and drive away. Fucking Alice in Wonderland and it was about to get even worse.

A few minutes passed, as my eyes continued to scan up and down the road for both potential threats and sources of help. Finally, a local police officer in a SUV pulled into the parking lot and got out of his car, asking me if I was okay. I told him

I had been on a long walk and didn't have my wallet or phone. He could see that I wasn't well and called an ambulance. I stood there covered in dirt and sweat as the EMTs arrived, still paranoid that I might be arrested at any moment.

Right off the bat, I felt like the EMTs were being strange as they took my vitals in the parking lot and inquired what had happened. My brain finally clicked into reality, and I came up with a story: I told them that my girlfriend and I had gotten into a bad argument so I got out of the car and walked. It sounded asinine, but what was I going to really say? They seemed to accept this story and I agreed to go to the hospital. Even though my brain had de-escalated from delusional to simply paranoid and I was no longer in a psychotic state, my fear center was still extremely active and guarded. As I was being escorted into the ambulance, my eyes landed on an immediate threat: Aileen's ex-husband was standing with an EMT about 10 feet away. I immediately asked the EMT next to me what that guy's name was, but he refused to answer. "Don't worry what his name is." I got strapped into the ambulance and they started an IV, my panic and fear rising with each passing minute.

On the way to the hospital, the EMTs were asking me a lot of questions that didn't seem to be related to what had occurred that day or information that the hospital would need about me. Things started to feel more and more 'off' and I felt trapped. I was facing backwards in the ambulance on a stretcher so I could see the traffic behind us, which seemed very strange to me. Suddenly, the driver initiated the privacy tint so I couldn't see who was behind us anymore. Then EMTs got quiet and they went towards the front of the ambulance. The privacy tint was turned off and I had a clear view directly into the van that was very close behind us: Aileen's ex-husband was driving it, looking rather pissed off and following so closely I don't know how he didn't hit us. A split second later, the tint was turned back on and the EMTs acted like nothing had occurred. I asked one question regarding the incident and was dismissed as if nothing had ever happened. I knew they were fucking with me; the screen had been down for only enough time for me to be completely certain about who was behind us. The funny part was he was a hick bitch who actually raped his best friends under age sister. Oh he was also a heroin addict so that moment he had was probably the crowning jewel of his life.

Lockwood

After the agonizing ride, we arrived at the hospital and I didn't know what to expect. Somehow, Aileen was already there waiting for me in the lobby, despite the fact that I had no phone to contact her and hadn't given the EMTs her information. Regardless, when compared to the day's events, she looked like safety to me and I refused the attending physician's recommendation that I be admitted given the state I was in and the psychotic episode I had just suffered. He was completely right, but my dopamine source was right there and willing to take me home, which sounded nice after being lost in the wilderness and psychologically tortured all day.

I think she expected me to be so grateful that I was going home alive and a free man that I would just put everything behind me, but that wasn't going to happen. When we got in the car, I immediately asked her why she told me that troopers were waiting to arrest me when she knew that wasn't true. She denied everything and insisted that she said nothing and I got out of the car on my own volition. I began to doubt myself, at this point aware that I had been psychotic for basically the entire day. Was she telling the truth, or had she really said what I heard her say? It certainly felt like something she would do, creating chaos to bring me further down and more dependent on only her.

She also denied everything about her ex-husband being involved that day, despite the fact that his presence was one of the things I was most certain about. I should have known right then and there by the way she was covering for him that they were more than just doing child visitation. I wouldn't have the truth confirmed until some time later, when Aileen's ex-mother-in-law needed to talk with my father regarding an unrelated issue. She confirmed to my dad that Aileen's ex had indeed been at that scene that day dressed as an EMT. What a bunch of hicks.

I had no recourse but to own the fact I had a psychotic episode and just absolutely embarrassed the shit out of myself in front of my wife's ex's entire town. In hindsight, I wasn't just running from the cops that day: I was practicing for when the day came that I would leave Aileen and never ever go back. While at that hospital, I had the option to be admitted and tell the staff I was in an abusive relationship. The thought crossed my mind and I weighed the options but wasn't fully ready to pull the trigger yet. Where would I go if I left? As is the point of an abuser's isolation tactics, I didn't feel like I had anyone in my life who I could ask for such a favor. There were angels in the wings sharpening their haloes, I just had to open my eyes to see.

*   *   *

Only a couple of weeks passed before I suffered another episode. I had just received a considerable amount of Adderall from a good friend and Aileen and I were headed to Jessica's house to take care of some business. Everything seemed normal as we arrived and exchanged friendly greetings. I was used to people being happy to see me; they usually are when they know you always travel with cocaine and pills. But Aileen was there to make a sale of her own to Jessica. The three of us stood in the kitchen and Aileen pulled out her stash. I was immediately struck by just how *many* pills she had in the bag, way more than her normal script.

Suspicious, I went back out of the kitchen and went to check my bag. Sure enough, the orange oval tablets that should have been there were now gone and replaced by a bunch of purple tablets I didn't recognize at all. Aileen had stolen my Adderall to sell to Jessica, and I started to get pissed off. I walked back over to the kitchen and angrily dumped the pills all over the counter, demanding an explanation from Aileen.

Aileen played dumb and denied everything. The proof was right there in front of her face: she had double the amount she should have had, and the ones I had earlier had been replaced. Jessica was no help; she was practically drooling over the huge bag of pills she had just purchased and, with a huge grin on her face, offered me a weak "Gee, Asher, that sucks". Neither of them seemed to realize how angry I was, so I stupidly grabbed a handful of the mystery pills and ate them to prove my point.

I blacked out and awoke in the passenger seat of the van with Aileen driving. I was completely incoherent and emotional; Aileen informed me that I was sobbing and generally making a spectacle of myself at Jessica's place, in full view of her kids. All I could think about was how awful I felt. I couldn't exactly pinpoint it at first, which only increased my anxiety level. What the fuck were those pills, and where did Aileen get them? *Did I just take a bunch of opiates?* How many did I take? How was I still breathing?

I tried to make sense of what just happened and looked outside to try and get my bearings. We were almost home. I felt like I was stuck in Jello. I opened my mouth to once again demand an explanation. Before I could get a word out, Aileen's cell started ringing on the overhead car Bluetooth. It was Jessica. The girls exchanged a few pleasantries as Aileen made the turn onto our street. "Don't you think we should prepare Asher for all the police waiting for him at your house?" Jessica's voice filled the van, tinged with a mocking tone.

Panic immediately took over. I flung open the car door and made it clear I was getting out no matter what. It was nighttime. Aileen slowed down enough for me to jump out of the car and start running, her voice disappearing behind me. I couldn't find anywhere immediately to hide; the street was completely residential. I sprinted through backyards in search of a dense patch of trees or an unlocked shed or *anything*. I kept glancing back towards the road as I ran, noticing a car with a very strange front-facing light cruising very slowly down the residential street.

A few yards away, I spotted a couple of conifer trees that looked close enough to each other to provide some cover. I dove in between them and did a full 360-degree assessment of my surroundings. A pack of pickup trucks drove past and I was sure they were hunting me. I couldn't stop seeing figures moving out of the corner of my eye. I suddenly realized just how far away from each other the trees I was hiding in actually were, and I knew I needed to keep moving.

I ran through the surrounding neighborhoods for what felt like hours hiding in garbage cans and pricker bushes before I found myself in a backyard with an enclosed treehouse. Upon investigation, I found that the only way into the treehouse was up a small ladder and through a trapdoor that opened inwards. I quickly scrambled up the ladder and inside, pulling the trapdoor closed behind me and lying down across it so no one could get in. Despite how sure I was that I could hear cops gathering beneath the tree to wait for me to come down, it was the safest I'd felt all day. I could finally catch my breath.

When I opened my eyes, I was immediately stung by long strips of blinding sun streaming in between the slats of the treehouse roof. *Did I fall asleep, or did I black out? Was it tomorrow, or had multiple days passed?* It was insanely hot and I was drenched in sweat and dehydrated. I needed to make a move. I sat up and was immediately struck by how hazy I felt between the dehydration, yesterday's adrenaline, and the remnants of the mystery pills in my system.

I opened the trapdoor and started to climb down. I looked down below to see squirt guns pointed at me and spraying water, but nothing was there when I finally reached the ground. I walked towards the front of the house and ran into a man coming towards me on the sidewalk. I think he asked me if I was okay, then another guy showed up. I started to feel even foggier than I did when I first woke up. The two men introduced themselves, and I was struck by how familiar their names sounded. I couldn't place where I had heard the names before. Old patients? Something more nefarious?

An ambulance materialized in front of me, and once again I found myself surrounded by suspicious EMTs. Their questions were odd and they seemed to be almost chiding me when I answered. I discovered that I was only one street over from my house, despite running for hours. I needed to stop talking and deal with this dehydration, ASAP. It seemed like the EMTs were purposely stalling to prolong my suffering, offering what seemed like an insincere apology because they were out of the "chilled" IV bags. What the fuck, who cares, just please set up the line! In an attempt to end the questioning and get treatment quicker, I gave them a bullshit story about getting drunk the night before and taking a walk. This "admission" necessitated a call to a state trooper, who arrived shortly.

Surprisingly, the cop seemed to be the only one who wasn't fucking with me. She asked me a few standard questions before determining that I just needed to be careful. Before we left, I had her call Aileen so she could follow us to the hospital. Still delusional, I was certain that I recognized the cars passing us on the highway.

To this day, I'm still not 100% certain what was in those pills that Aileen switched with my Adderall. She continued to deny everything and act like I was crazy. I also could never figure out why Jessica went along with the charade and made the call in the van that day. But when I de-escalated from the psychotic episode and tried to piece together what had happened, one thing was clear: I had once again been made to look like a fool by Aileen. Looking back, it is so obvious how she was trying to tear me to pieces and I stayed despite it all. Addiction had rendered me blind; I was so sure I would be able to get a handle on the situation but she made it impossible. She didn't want me to stabilize because, in her mind, it meant I would give her less attention or maybe even connect the dots that she was the one trying to sabotage my life. The more paranoid and ill and afraid of the outside world I became, the more I would isolate myself at home with her.

Aileen's need for attention was all-consuming; it was like my need for external validation but multiplied by a hundred. Nothing I could do was ever enough and all the ground I gave up to her only made her keep moving the finish line further and further away. At her behest, I had pushed away everyone who was close to me, including my family. After she pulled the stunt where she discharged all of my patients via email without my permission, my practice was in complete shambles. I had no money coming in, to the point where I couldn't even keep my prepaid cell phone in service consistently. Any attempt I made at reestablishing my practice was undone almost immediately. I spent a great deal of the summer of 2022 isolated in the house with Aileen, just like she always wanted, sitting at home like an ornament and starring in the videos she would post on social media to show how "in love" we were (the lesser of two evils when compared with the defamation and threats she had posted before). I think that if given the chance, her ultimate dream would be to see me bound and gagged in her basement forever. Or in jail.

That summer, it finally dawned on me why Aileen's ex-husband seemed so happy when he shook my hand the first time I met him way back when. His mom had warned my dad that Aileen had drained the life from her ex and that she'd do it to me, too. It was true; she turned him into a husk. When her focus shifted off of him and onto me, it released him from a curse. He was happy to be replaced because it meant that he was finally free of the all-consuming sisyphean task of feeding an attention monster that could never be satiated. Sure, she kept him around for hookups every now and then, but the one caught squarely in the crossfire of her chaos was *me*. If only I had recognized it at the time.

My Ride or Dies

As the summer progressed, I started to get fed up with everything in a way that felt more actionable and *real*. Aileen had me pinned, but she got too greedy and it was too much to ignore. A year earlier, I was making like $5000.000 a week, working on Aces Bay with my friends, driving a Mercedes, and planning to reopen a brick-and-mortar practice. Now, I had nothing. I couldn't keep control of an email account for longer than 24 hours, had no way for patients to book, not a dollar to my name, no cell phone (the cheap prepaid flip phones I would buy kept mysteriously disappearing or would run out of funds because of how broke I was), and an old van with no gas. That's what she wanted, a slave that answered just her. That's what she had done to her ex-husband except he had no means to escape and imploded on heroin. I was simply not going to do that.

I made several trips to stay with Michael and his family for a few days at a time over that summer. I had to sneak out early in the morning before she was awake so she didn't see me taking the van. They never made me feel crazy or like I was imposing; I was always welcomed with no questions asked by his whole family. Michael would get me some cell phone minutes and sit with me for hours and hours, untangling accounts and passwords and helping me get a booking platform online so I could start working again.

Each time, without fail, Aileen would always get a hold of me after two or three days and ask when I was coming home. When that happened, I took it as a sign that whatever insanity or fight that had occurred before my departure was forgiven and I would return home. In reality, Aileen's perception that I had "abandoned" her was more than she could accept, and she would become desperate to regain control of the situation. When I would return home, her excitement at my presence and attention was usually stronger than any desire she had to torture me as punishment for leaving. Aileen would be on her best behavior for a few days, lulling me into a false sense of security that I mistook for peace.

Whenever I decided to go back home, Michael never tried to stop me; he knew me well enough to know that I had to come to the conclusion on my own if it was going to stick for real. But each time, I gained a little bit more clarity and insight (even if it took me a week or two to realize it). Michael had a way of getting a point across without hitting me over the head with it or being patronizing (and getting to sleep, eat, and live peacefully for a couple of days at a time definitely didn't hurt).

I left Michael's house for the third and last time that summer with a bizarre optimism. I knew I was done with feeling like I was letting life just happen to me. I was ready to take control. I convinced myself that Aileen wasn't actually the problem, she was just acting out because of the stress of CPS and losing her kids. Maybe I really wasn't giving her enough attention. I bid adieu to Michael and his family and started the journey home to Aileen, filled with a renewed desire to be the perfect husband in order to fix our relationship. I could do it! In a world of complete insanity, it felt nice to honestly believe that I had the power to repair everything that felt wrong with my life.

I got on the road as the summer sun was starting to set. I had made up my mind, felt like I had finally figured something out, and I knew there was someone special I needed to share the news with. *"Hello?"* It had been almost a month since I had last heard Elle's voice. I wasn't surprised when she picked up right away; I don't think she had ever missed one of my calls. I was sober and felt clear-headed and I could tell by her voice that she was happy to hear from me.

I updated her on what I had been up to the past few weeks and shared my epiphany with her. She admitted that she had been worried about me since I went dark and often wondered how I was doing. She was happy to hear that I was focused on my sobriety and family and her approval only reaffirmed the decision in my mind. She took it well, the conversation flowed easily, and she kept me company for hours. I told her how appreciative I was for the things she'd done for me and offered a quick blanket apology for the general insanity that had occurred. At one point, she told me that she always dreamed about having this kind of conversation with me. It was the closure that I was hoping for.

I made it back to Bergen a little before midnight. I let her know that I only had a few minutes left to chat. In response, she asked me when she could expect to see or hear from me again. I was confused and surprised – the entire point of my call to her was to share my decision to commit to my marriage and do everything right by Aileen. I assumed she had read between the lines earlier and understood that it meant that I needed to go into this with a pure soul. Even though the relationship between myself and Elle was far from an affair in our hearts, it couldn't continue.

"Oh." Her voice changed, becoming quieter and weaker. I couldn't tell if she was about to start crying. I made the turn onto my street. Words came out of her, a question, but I couldn't engage. I didn't have time, I was approaching the duplex. Something was in the window. I got closer and saw it was Aileen – despite the late hour, and my arrival being a complete surprise, she was standing in front of the window as if she was expecting me. Perched like a bird of prey, motionless in the darkness. Our street was so quiet and I knew that the massive, hollow van amplified phone conversations on speakerphone to the point where they could be heard inside the entryway of the house. If Aileen heard that I was talking to Elle, it would cause a fight that would threaten my attempts to fix everything. I repeated that I HAD to go, now, I had just arrived home. I hung up the call as I pulled into the driveway, abruptly silencing the confused stream of questions that came squeaking out of Elle.

I went inside to start my new life as a sober loving husband and father.

*   *   *

I don't think I need to say that my new lease on life didn't last long. Within days of my arrival at home, Aileen had done everything in her power to remind me of exactly why I left in the first place. At Michael's house, with the relief of having all my clinical accounts straightened out, far away from Aileen, it was easy to convince myself that she was simply a lonely wife and a sad mother without her kids and I just needed to be more understanding and affectionate and present and it would fix everything. I was sincere and gave it my best effort, doing everything right. I spent my first several days back at home doing nothing but showering her with attention as an apology for leaving.

She barely took notice. After a day or two, it seemed like she was only happy that I came home because she once again had someone to subject to non-stop criticism, insults, accusations, and orchestrated drama. It was a week before I couldn't take it anymore. I woke up hours before I knew Aileen would be awake and found myself in Elle's parking lot a little before 7:00 a.m. I dialed her number and I could tell by her voice when she answered that I had woken her up. "Are you at home? I'm in your parking lot right now." Within seconds, her front door opened and she sleepily stumbled into the parking lot and up into the passenger seat of the van. I remember thinking how amazing it was that she was always there for me at the drop of a hat, no questions asked. Yes, I was very much falling in love with her. Again.

"Ok actually, thank God that you're here. I'm so happy to see you, because last week has been awful. I literally was on a dating app and went on a date with a stranger last night for the first time ever and it was *awful* and I literally never want to do it again. I don't even want to date, I just wanted to like, be respectful of your decision and try to move on but everyone out their sucks." The words tumbled out of her mouth the second her butt hit the seat of the car. She was wearing a dress and black tights and sneakers, obviously having fallen asleep in her clothes from the night before. "I really think this guy just didn't want to eat dinner alone. I kept trying to talk to him about his business and his like, sublimation printing machine and it was very clear he was not into it and it was awkward and weird. Even though I *literally* put front and center in my Tinder bio, 'I really want to talk about your business', I think he didn't know I was serious? Please tell me I don't have to do that anymore and that's why you're here."

Her words hurt in a way I wasn't expecting; I never considered the possibility that she could have been swept off her feet by some guy and gone from my life forever. What if I had waited a day to make this visit? A week? I avoided directly answering her question about if my visit meant that she was off the market, but if she noticed, she didn't say anything. It was clear she was just happy to see me. Her rambling filled the car and immediately, I was smiling again. Even with last night's makeup under her eyes, she was cute. I noticed she had gotten a haircut since I had last seen her, she had cut it to a little past her shoulders and added bangs. I told her I liked her outfit and that her new haircut was "sassy." She was acting like a teenager with a crush, just like usual when we saw each other again after a while. Sometimes it annoyed me, but today, I found it endearing.

Adderall and Other False Prophets

Without getting into it too much, I confided that Aileen was back to her endless pursuit of filling my life with misery. "I think everyone knows that you were never the problem," Elle reminded me as I pulled out of her lot. I took her to the only place that was open this early on a weekday: Walmart. We walked around the store while talking. When that got old, we walked around the grocery store. The conversation between us came as easily as I remembered, and being with her felt so natural. With Aileen, I was constantly policing myself and walking on eggshells and still always found myself getting insulted or screamed at or worse. Nothing I did was ever right. With Elle, I could just...be myself, and have a conversation with her, and that was the right thing, without needing to try or contort myself into an impossible expectation.

It was a beautiful day, and we went back to the van. I started driving, but instead of leaving the parking lot I just pulled into a space in the most out-of-the-way section, facing nothing but a chain link fence, some trees, and the back of a commercial building. She turned to ask me what we were doing and I immediately pulled her into a kiss. It had been so long that I forgot how right it felt. I took her to St. Theresa's Cemetery and drove past the rows of headstones into a small clearing surrounded by trees, overlooking a cliff. I always found that place so peaceful. I felt safe there.

I parked, and we sat in the grass and looked down at the cliff and continued talking. It was easy to be emotionally open and vulnerable with her without fear that it would be weaponized against me. I talked about my sons and wanting to do better for them and missing my friends and the normal life I had before everything happened. She listened.

Aileen checked in with me via text every so often. The excuse I left on a note to explain my early-morning absence was that I was meeting up with my boy Warren to get info on state jobs I could apply for. I knew she'd be happy with this; if I was going to work, she wanted me at a 9:00 a.m.-5:00 p.m. "Running a business" took too much of my time and attention away from her, according to her, and I knew she'd be excited if I told her that the coworkers at these jobs were likely to be only other men and no women. Plus, Warren was a powerful attorney in the area (in addition to being male, obviously), and therefore Aileen would allow me to spend a few hours with him. But I knew better than to push my luck, and soon I figured it would be smart to drive Elle back to her apartment.

She ran inside and printed off pages of relevant state job listings for me to bring home so that the day wouldn't be a complete lie. We continued talking for a bit, with the conversation turning deeper and deeper as morning turned to early afternoon. I didn't want to leave, but Aileen had gone eerily silent and I wanted to keep everything as drama-free as possible. I left Elle with the question of who'd she want to play her when they make my life into a movie before returning home to Aileen.

I had come home so early that she bought everything, with the printouts lending an added touch of realism. The day continued uneventfully until later that night. I opened my laptop and went on Amazon to try and buy a new package of soap or something. When the page loaded, I was surprised to see that the login fields were autofilled with the email and password for my Amazon business account, which I hadn't used in months, instead of the login credentials for my personal Amazon account. Out of curiosity, I clicked the Sign In button and was surprised to see that the credentials worked.

It was odd that this account was logged in here; I went through laptops so often that I knew for certain that this computer was purchased long after the last time I accessed my Amazon business account. In fact, I had completely lost access to the account months ago and wrote it off entirely. The whole thing was suspicious. I navigated to the account history out of curiosity and saw a seemingly endless list of unfamiliar transactions. I scrolled through row after row of massive expensive purchases charged to my card on file and what were clearly fraudulent returns, expensive things that I knew she hadn't actually returned.

Confusion turned to revulsion as I started to make sense of what I was seeing: Aileen was using this Amazon account, linked directly to my psychiatry business's EIN, to run a return scam. She would use my card to buy something expensive (like multiple giant chicken coops for the backyard), initiate a return, but keep the item. For some reason, the Amazon sellers kept issuing refunds anyway. Instead of the money going back to the original payment method (again, my debit card), she was getting the refunds issued as Amazon gift cards, which I then assumed she used on her own personal Amazon account to buy more crap. This had gone on for months, a year, maybe longer. I didn't need to add up the total amount to know it had crossed the threshold into serious fraud.

I pulled a couple months of printed bank statements out of my nearby filing cabinet to confirm. Sure enough, the purchases on the account matched up with Amazon charges on the bank statements. No refunds were ever issued to my bank account despite the fact that she used my money to buy everything. She kept all the refunds for herself while using my business info to commit fraud. I was shocked and felt betrayed. I printed out the Amazon order history as proof and continued combing through the statements. For months, I kept ordering new debit cards that would never arrive and was constantly locked out of my online banking account. The statements began to paint a picture: every time I would order a new debit card, she would grab it from the mail, activate it and set a pin, and make odd withdrawals in amounts that were different from the ones I would make. Since I wasn't in possession of the "active" card, I couldn't use the card number to regain access to my account. She would stop the withdrawals for long enough that the transaction would be buried by deposits from the payment processor I used for patient appointments and allow me to receive maybe every third or fourth new debit card I requested. By the time I got the card, I usually only checked that I had enough in the account to score an eight ball and I didn't catch her stealing.

I scanned through everything quickly, feeling nauseous. I stopped counting when I got to around $10,000.00 that she had stolen from me. I knew she messed with my stuff but I never expected that it was this blatant. She was straight-up just stealing money from me. I took her out of the strip club, I let her be a stay-at-home mom like she claimed she wanted, I paid all the bills, I paid off all her debts and fixed her credit while mine continued to get worse, I took her out to dinner constantly, I took her on vacations, I gave her *everything* even a 2 carat $22,000.00 diamond ring. I didn't even expect her to help out answering the phones anymore! The entire time, she was just brazenly stealing from me.

In shock, I went upstairs and confronted her about my Amazon account. She brushed it off and said I told her she could use my card on Amazon. I was speechless. Buying a few small things on Amazon here and there like a normal person was one thing. Throwing myself and my business under the bus for thousands of dollars of fraud, spending my money and keeping the refunds for herself was completely different. Her excuse didn't even make any sense. She had access to my current personal Amazon account, the one we used for normal purchases. If she wasn't trying to hide anything, why wouldn't she use that one instead of one she thought I no longer had access to? Disgusted and devastated, I returned to the basement. She was a vampire in every sense of the word and I couldn't even look at her.

Over the last few months, I barely had time to catch my breath and process her most recent betrayal before the next one became evident. I was still reeling from the last one: after returning from Michael's house, I discovered that Aileen's father had given her a car because I had taken the van with me. This "gift" left me in total disbelief. I had spent the last seven months without a vehicle, and Aileen saw me waste probably hundreds of hours of time exploring every avenue available to secure a vehicle with my abysmal credit. She saw me get scammed out of several thousand dollars by one of Jessica's friends who worked at a car dealership. The entire time, she knew her dad had an extra vehicle sitting around, just waiting for her to ask for it. Was I even supposed to find out about the car? If I hadn't shown up unannounced, did she plan to bring it back to him so I never found out and she could continue to have the opportunity to hold "her" car (paid for by me, of course), the van, over my head as our only vehicle? I took having a nice car for granted for most of my adult life and now faced a situation where my having access to *any* vehicle, for any length of time, the bare minimum of autonomy, was just too much of a threat for her.

As soon as the sun rose, my instinct was to call Elle. As soon as she picked up, I was sobbing again. The only words I could get out were *"she took everything from me."* She had no idea what I was talking about, and I tried my best to explain the Amazon stuff.

"Do you want to come over again?" she asked, and I once again found myself in the van on my way to her. By the time I arrived, I had composed myself a bit. She was already waiting in the parking lot for me with a box of Boston Cream donuts. She got into the car and I passed her the printouts from Amazon and the bank. I immediately got upset again. Our entire relationship, every time Aileen fucked me over, I wrote it off as the childish lashing-out of a traumatized borderline when she felt abandoned. But this discovery left me rethinking everything. Maybe she was never impulsive at all. Maybe everything she had ever done to hurt me was as calculated and organized as the sophisticated return scam.

Elle tried to make sense of what she was looking at as I tried again to explain in between bites of donut. "So...this is fucked up," she finally announced after flipping through the pages. "I have no idea why Amazon would keep issuing these refunds if she wasn't sending anything back. I didn't even know you could get a refund through a method other than the original form of payment?" None of it made any sense, yet it was all there in black and white.

Since the whole thing was vaguely computer adjacent, I wondered if Nathan would have any idea how Aileen did it or if I was likely to get in trouble for her misdeeds. I dialed his number and put it on speaker. In between rings, I tried to remember if things had ended on bad terms the last time we spoke. My brain gave me nothing, but my gut told me yes. Fortunately, just like everyone else who was even remotely close to me at any point since I first met Aileen, Nathan hated her in a way that ran deeper than whatever he and I may have had going on.

He finally answered, and Elle and I took turns explaining what I had found. "I doubt she knows someone at Amazon. I dunno. I've kind of heard of this. I think there's a thing where sometimes if you say the item arrives damaged, the seller doesn't want it back? Especially if it's something heavy that would cost them a ton in shipping. If they think it's broken, they can't sell it again anyway. But Amazon catches on if you do it too much, especially if it's a new account and you immediately start trying to return everything. If the account is seasoned and has a normal-looking history of purchases without issue you can probably get away with it for longer. Have you tried slapping her in the face with a moldy steak?" Good to see Nathan hadn't lost his way with words.

All of that stuff made sense, but I think what I really wanted was a more personal answer. The entire time, was I nothing but an easy mark to Aileen? Did I exist to her only as a resource to bleed dry? I cycled through emotions; hurt, angry, sad, betrayed, angry again. Elle could read it on my face and she reached over from the passenger seat to give me a hug. I wasn't sure where to go from there.

We drove around, and she let me vent. As opposed to the day before when I was on my best behavior, I left that morning without leaving a note and hadn't yet texted Aileen. She would be waking up to an empty house, and I knew it could go one of two ways: she was either going to be ripshit pissed at me and there would be hell to pay when I returned, or she would realize how badly she messed up and slip into her dumb cutesy baby persona and let me get away with being gone for the day.

As a distraction, we took the van through the carwash and dried it by hand. I suddenly remembered again about the free car from her dad and started to get upset. I decided that, since I was paying for the van, it should be "my car" now that she had another one. First order of business: peeling all of Aileen's stupid tacky stickers off the back. Unfortunately, that didn't kill as much time as I had hoped and I wasn't sure where to go after that. Hours had gone by, and noon came and went with still no word from Aileen. She had to be awake by now. She had a special talent of somehow being able to tell when I was gone even while she was still asleep, which made her wake up even earlier. I started to fear for the worst and didn't want to even go home. Instead, I asked Elle if she wanted to do something fun that night.

"Like what, the drive-in or something? I think that could be cool," Elle suggested. That wasn't really what I had in mind, but she seemed genuinely excited about it. She could be such a dork sometimes.

I forced out a laugh. "I don't know. Do you think I should check with Aileen and see if I'm allowed to have fun with you?" I tried to joke.

"Yeah, definitely don't do that. I don't want to die today." Elle said, forcing a smile. She could tell I was preoccupied. We were aimlessly driving on the highway at this point, and I tried to decide what to do. Aileen's anger had been escalating lately, so if I went home, I wasn't sure what I'd be walking into. I couldn't tell if I should reach out to her first. Her silence was either a sign that everything was fine or that she was waiting behind the front door with a knife.

I drove around with the windows down, and the stack of papers I brought with me that morning started fluttering around. Elle scrambled to gather them all and stuffed them under the flap of her shoulder bag to keep them together. We ended up in the mall parking lot, standing outside in the sun. Elle tried to engage me in conversation, but my mind was elsewhere. I finally decided to investigate the situation and shot Aileen a text. I kept it very light, asking how her day was and using my romantic nickname for her. It was a peace offering of sorts. Immediately, my phone started ringing. I motioned for Elle to keep quiet and I answered the call on speaker.

I braced myself for screaming and was caught off-guard by her sugary-sweet tone. She told me that she decided to make some Doordash deliveries for extra money for us, and she was having a profitable day. I listened to her bullshit story about how she was waiting for an order at a restaurant and met a group of other Doordashers. They were all women, and their husbands all took care of all their bills just like I did for her, and they only made deliveries so they had extra spending money for purses and whatever. Then they all compared their engagement rings, and Aileen's was the biggest, and she told them all how I was a big-time nurse practitioner and how lucky she was. Oh, and luckily she had totally figured out the "$10,000.00 Amazon thing" and it was all a big misunderstanding and everything was actually fine!

Every aspect of it was a lie, obviously, but none of that mattered. The important thing was that she was extending an obvious olive branch to me. She wasn't angry that I snuck out without telling her or accusing her of stealing. I told her that I had been at the library applying for jobs all morning and at CarMax all afternoon looking to see if I could trade the van for something nicer for us, but that I was actually on my way home now and I couldn't wait to see her. Obviously unaware that she was on speaker or that Elle was with me, she ended the call by saying that she was on her period so it would have to be a 210 night, lucky me (Long Island Slang).

Elle was straining not to roll her eyes while also holding her breath, trying to stay completely silent in case Aileen somehow sensed her presence through the phone. Always anxious, she waited a good several seconds after we hung up to start talking, just in case. "That's such a lie. No one does Doordash for that, let alone a whole group of them in one place?"

"Yeah, I know," I said, hopping into the car and slamming the key into the ignition. "I gotta drop you off and get home."

"Yeah," her voice was tinged with disappointment that didn't even register to me at the time. "So, I guess this means no drive-in?" She forced a smile and I peeled out of the mall parking lot.

"What? Yeah, no. She just gave me a get-out-of-jail-free card." I sped down the highway towards Elle's apartment. "She let everything slide, and I get to spend the night in bed with my wife, not running around all night finding trouble. It was a peace offering." I felt nothing but relief. Maybe I had the right idea after leaving Michael's after all, and I only needed to follow certain rules in order to keep the peace all the time.

I barely came to a full stop in front of Elle's apartment. *Please don't try to kiss me or pull any chick shit*, I mentally pleaded. She grabbed her stuff and got out. "I gotta go, but I'll call you soon," I offered before starting to pull away.

"Wait! Your papers?" She pulled the stack of Amazon and bank printouts out of the front of her bag from earlier and tried to hand them to me through the window.

"I don't want them; you can throw them out!" I called, waving once out the window as I drove away.

*   *   *

I woke up from an accidental nap that evening to find the house empty and Aileen's new car gone. The whiteboard where we used to leave each other's notes was empty, and I had no texts or calls. It was a little odd, but I tried not to jump to conclusions after she had been so "understanding" towards me that day. My call to her phone immediately went to voicemail, as if her phone was dead or I was blocked. I fired off a quick text and waited for a reply. Several minutes went by with no response.

I tried to see if any of her more ostentatious outfits were missing from the closet in an attempt to piece together where she might have gone. Nothing stood out to me, but I did find her clown makeup kit open and strewn about in front of the mirror. I thought about where she might go. The Electric Co.? Probably not, it was the middle of the week and there would be hardly anyone there. It'd also be odd for her to go alone after we spent the afternoon and early evening on good terms.

Had she been hanging out with anyone lately? Maybe Jessica? It wouldn't be the first time I caught them sneaking around together at night. But this was different. Something felt wrong, and worry took hold within me. I fired off a desperate text to Jessica. I was distrustful of her after the obvious recent incidents, but she was also helping us with CPS stuff. I followed up the text with *I'm worried.* so she knew this wasn't the usual "Asher and Aileen drama".

I paced around our bedroom, darting to the window every time a car passed by to see if it was her. I couldn't tell if it was smarter for me to stay home in case she showed up or leave the house to look for her. It had been a little while now and my anxiety increased exponentially with each call I made to her that went unanswered. Suddenly, my phone lit up and I pounced on it. Just fucking Jessica. *No idea where she is. Just make sure no one shows up here tonight.*

The old familiar fear of abandonment wrapped around me and I started to panic. I couldn't decide what to do next and worst-case scenarios flashed through my brain. After a few more desperate calls to Aileen went to voicemail, I tried to run through my options. I couldn't call the cops; she hadn't been gone long enough and Jessica had hammered into our heads that we really needed to try to avoid any police activity for the good of our CPS case after everything that had happened. *Who could I trust to help me find her?* Even though the events from earlier in the day seemed so long ago, I immediately thought of how willing Elle had been to help out. I dialed her number.

She could hear the fear in my voice and was immediately willing to help. She took the situation seriously, and I asked if she could try and find out if there were any performances or events going on that night that might have grabbed Aileen's attention. Elle tried to talk me down in between reading off local event calendars and looking for karaoke nights. She checked Aileen's social media for any clues, but she hadn't posted anything public recently. I wondered if Nathan would have any ideas for seeing if she had left any other online clues or knew of some way to tell if her phone was even on.

Lockwood

It was late, but Elle offered to pick up Nathan and come up to Bergen. She was driving her ex-boyfriend's car (she still hadn't been able to afford getting her car fixed and out of the tow lot from June), which Aileen wouldn't recognize. I gave Elle a description of the car Aileen was driving, the one from her dad, and she agreed to check the parking lots in town. I would stay at home if Aileen showed up.

After about 45 minutes, a text from Elle came through. A picture of Aileen's car, at the back of the local Walmart parking lot. Immediately, my fear and worry started to warp into realization that there was no danger and Aileen was just up to no good. They told me that the car was empty and no one else was parked near it. The store was still open but would be closing shortly, at midnight, and they didn't want to hang around and risk a confrontation with Aileen. I asked them to come pick me up.

By the time we got back to the lot, the store had closed and Aileen's car was gone. Even though she still hadn't replied, I fired off a text as an alibi in case she got home before me and wondered why I hadn't taken the van: I noticed she was out and went to look for her in a cab so we would only need to drive one car home.

We drove past the duplex and her car still wasn't there, so she clearly hadn't gone home immediately after leaving the parking lot. We checked the local bars, Elle and Nathan staying in the car far away from the entrance while I scanned the parking lot and went inside to look for her. Even in a crisis situation, I knew that the absolute worst thing I could do in Aileen's eyes was reach out to Elle.

We couldn't find her. It was a weeknight, and even the bars were closing by now. Elle was almost back at the duplex to drop me off when my phone suddenly lit up. It was Aileen, asking if I was at home. My heart rate immediately spiked. If Aileen was already at home, I absolutely could not risk her seeing me getting dropped off by Elle and Nathan. Even though Elle was driving a car that Aileen wouldn't recognize, there was a huge chance that she would be outside waiting for me. Time for a change of plans.

I had Elle pull off into a side street and drop me off in the parking lot of an auto repair shop that always had their parking lot lights turned on. I was maybe a quarter of a mile from the duplex but called a cab anyway so my story matched. She was home by the time I arrived, seemingly oblivious to the fact that I was becoming angry. I couldn't believe that she let me spend the night worried, sick and panicking as part of her attention-seeking game.

I immediately started questioning where she had been all night and why she didn't answer me. I told her I saw her car in the Walmart parking lot. She told me she was just taking a nap in her car and therefore couldn't hear her phone ringing nonstop from my calls. She didn't have an explanation for why she had left without telling me so she could take a nap in a parking lot, or where she had gone after that. Nothing about her story was adding up, but I didn't have proof. That was how she operated; no matter how obvious it was that she was lying, the burden of proof was always on me. *Prove it.*

While I never got a real explanation out of Aileen about the events of that night, I was able to eventually come to my own conclusion. Her behavior had all the 'tells' of a cheating episode, but her outfit was the dead giveaway. She wasn't overly done up, so I knew that it couldn't be one of the older guys she messed around with for money. It was someone she was comfortable with. Since they met up in a parking lot, it must have been someone who couldn't afford even one night in a hotel. And it was late at night in the middle of the week, so it was probably someone without a normal job. Every sign pointed directly to her ex-husband. My thought was that the two of them were in his car in the Walmart parking lot, close enough to her car that she could keep an eye on it.

The timing of everything made sense. After Elle texted me the picture Nathan took of Aileen's car in the parking lot, they made the seven-minute drive to go pick me up. Aileen might have seen Nathan standing by her car, but she wouldn't have recognized the car Elle was driving and probably had no idea it was them. By the time we got to the lot, Aileen's car was gone, and I think she may have circled the duplex at first, trying to figure out if I was home or not. Even though she was ignoring my texts, she was definitely reading them as they came in. She made sure I was far enough away from the house in my search that she'd finally have time to park at home, go inside, and take a shower so there was no physical evidence of her escapade. She knew I'd be worried sick and go out looking for her, but I think it threw her off that I didn't take the van; she had probably been planning to rely on whether it was in the driveway to determine if I was home or not.

Lockwood

When I figured it out, I didn't confront her about it. As she always did when I caught her stepping out, she played nice for a few days and I wanted to keep the peace. Whenever things were calm for a few blessed days, I wanted to believe it would last forever. Unfortunately, she would always get bored and start looking for ways to inject chaos, and it wasn't too long until I found myself seeking a way out once again.

Living Clean Dying Quietly

By the end of August 2022, our lease at the duplex was circling the drain – just like everything else between Aileen and myself. We were in a bad place. The rental was a warzone and I was in the trenches. Most days began with accusations and ended with screaming matches, shattered picture frames, and her peeling out of the driveway in a rage. We were toxic, volatile, and once again being shown the door via a terminated lease (no surprise there). I'd lost count of how many landlords had tossed us out. This was just another burned bridge.

She had plans to move into her widowed father's house with him, but I wasn't sure where I was going to live. She made it clear that I wasn't invited, but truthfully, I had no desire to live with her at her father's. I'd only met the man once, five years earlier. Based on how he was throwing vehicles and thousands of dollars at her, I could only imagine the lies she had told him about me.

Regardless of where I was going, I needed to have everything packed and out of the duplex by the end of the month. I hate moving more than anything. It's a special kind of hell, packing up your entire life into boxes and pretending it's just "stuff." In the midst of all the cardboard box chaos, with every last one of my earthly possessions scattered throughout the house as if a bomb detonated, Aileen came at me. I was so exhausted from the constant stream of verbal bile she spat at me, and at the same time, so overstimulated by the stress of packing and the looming threat of homelessness. I just needed everything to stop so I could think and breathe for a minute.

I ducked into the bathroom and did what I told myself I wouldn't: I called Elle out of the blue and implored her in a whisper to call me an Uber. Within ten minutes, the car pulled up and I just...went outside and got in it. I knew there would be hell to pay from Aileen, but if I didn't get a few days of peace *now*, things would get much worse for me. My mental and physical health were already the worst they'd ever been, and every day was darker than the last. I really wasn't sure what would happen to me if I didn't get out for a little bit.

I slept off the abuse for a few days at Elle's apartment before asking her to help me get my practice back up and running. She woke me up several times a day to bring me food and remind me to take my meds and she agreed to help me get the work stuff straightened out. I asked for a change of scenery, so she booked a secluded Airbnb in Vermont for a night. On the way back, I nodded out on the highway in Massachusetts while driving her car (completely sober, just exhausted) and slammed into a guardrail, denting the entire length of the passenger side of the car and eventually getting pulled over after a concerned driver saw what happened and called it in. Despite the accident, the time I spent with Elle was peaceful and put me in a better headspace.

I'll spare you the details, but by the end of the week, I repaid Elle's hospitality by leaving about a third of my belongings (including a broken 70-inch TV) in her living room, making up an excuse to have her drive me to meet Aileen "just for an hour or two," and then sending her an email where I made fun of her and told her Aileen was about to give me a 210. Not my classiest moment.

Oh, and I ended up being right about the "hell to pay" part with Aileen. I wouldn't find out until much, much later, but she had spent the days I was with Elle filing false reports about me to basically every government agency with an online submission form – the Department of Health, the DEA, the state troopers, you name it. Despite how busy that must have kept her, she somehow found time to fuck her ex-husband, create a profile on a sugar daddy website, chat up a guy on the site, and then roll her dad's car after hitting another vehicle on a two-hour drive to meet him.

Completely unaware of Aileen's CVS-receipt-length list of betrayals, I wanted to make up with her. So, tail between my legs, I did what addicts and codependents do best – I came crawling back, hoping for an invitation to stay at her father's with her. She seemed to agree, and I assumed this meant that she talked about it with him. The movers had already brought everything of mine from the duplex that I couldn't fit at Elle's apartment to Aileen's fathers, which seemed like a good sign. On September 3, 2022, she confidently walked me into her father's house. I relaxed, thinking of the warm welcome I was about to receive. I even let myself feel a sliver of hope; maybe this would finally be the place where we could get our shit together, things could be stable, peaceful, happy...

Adderall and Other False Prophets

"I don't think so," he said flatly as soon as I walked in, eyes glued to the TV. He was sitting in the den, drinking scotch and watching the Red Sox lose again. The dog growled at me like it knew everything I'd ever done. His coldness caught me completely off guard. Genuinely out of options, I pictured myself hitchhiking to Connecticut with nothing but a duffle bag.

But this was the guy who seemed to have no shortage of cash or sensible vehicles to throw at Aileen to keep her quiet, and she knew that his "no" never really meant "no". The three of us had a discussion, and I tried to ignore the disconcerting smile plastered across her face the entire time. Eventually, he agreed to let me stay for a trial period. Relieved, I gave him a hug and thanked him. To be honest, I understood where he was coming from at first. He didn't know me from Adam, and all he had to go on over the past five years were the bizarre and concerning CPS reports – most, if not all, submitted by Aileen in fits of rage.

Aileen gave me a tour of the house, and it was obvious it hadn't been cleaned in a long time (probably not since his wife died a few years ago). Finally, we got to our quarters in the basement. The smell of mildew hit me halfway down the stairs. Then I saw all the boxes and old furniture and just...*crap*, everywhere. Oh, great, the chickens were down here too, for some reason. The place was very bleak, but I went along with it. In my mind, I had nowhere else to go. Most of my stuff was here, so I felt like I had to stay, too.

Life at her dad's house was strange. Aileen regressed, acting like a bratty kid until her father corrected her as if she was an actual child (which she would respond to, for the most part). He would hand her giant wads of cash constantly, for no good reason, as if it was an allowance she was entitled to. She considered any money acquired this way to be entirely hers and hers alone to blow on pointless discretionary shit. Startup costs to get my practice up and running again so we could move towards independence? Nope! Money to put aside for a car, since she totaled the one her dad gave her? Not a chance. The whole situation made no sense to me, and I don't think it ever will. I pulled him aside once and told him, gently, that he should ask for receipts. She was bleeding him dry, and he didn't really care; strange.

We got settled in and tried to establish some sort of routine. I was able to gradually start building my practice back up again, reaching out to patients as soon as I was able to get a booking platform online again. With no car between us (thanks to the last two she'd totaled) we started looking. Eventually, we found a used Honda Accord. It was clean, ran well, and didn't break the budget. Against all odds, we were approved for financing. Things almost felt normal for a few minutes.

It was only a couple of weeks until any dreams I had of this being a "fresh start" were shattered. One afternoon, as autumn leaves skittered across the driveway, I popped the hood of the car to check something. There, tangled beneath the frame, were unfamiliar wires. Not part of the engine. Not standard. My mind instantly flooded with suspicion. Was it a tracker? A wiretap? A bomb?

I called the cops. They came out, poked around, and said, "Not an explosive." Like that was supposed to be reassuring. Paranoia crept in like a fog that got thicker by the day until I couldn't see clearly. Why couldn't anything ever be simple or safe? Why couldn't I just be allowed to exist in peace? I walked across the street and asked the neighbor if he had any camera footage of our driveway. He checked. Nothing. No cars. No visitors. Just the still frame of me checking under the hood.

The wires continued to haunt me. To me, it had to be Nathan or Elle. Whoever did it must have been able to trim out the footage from the neighbor's camera feed. It didn't matter that neither of them knew anything about cars. It didn't matter that I had just seen Elle a month ago, and she had done nothing but try her best to make me as comfortable, happy, and healthy as possible. Logic had left the building. I spent nights parked by the window, eyes fixed on the road like a sentry. Every pair of headlights made my heart thump. I waited for a car to stop. It never did.

Running on fumes, eventually I cracked and fired off a scorched-earth email to both Elle and Nathan. It was filled with the most bizarre accusations to date and dripped with hatred. I told them to stay the hell away from me, my wife, my practice, my property, my life. As always, Aileen was right over my shoulder, getting me more worked up as I wrote the email. Fanning the flames, loving the circus. She always did. Chaos was her love language.

A week passed and I slowly regained the ability to think straight. I took one last look under the hood and traced the wires to their source. My stomach sank as I realized what I was looking at for the first time. The "surveillance wires" were nothing more than remnants of a goddamn tow package. The Accord had a hitch. Of course. Shame burned my face as I remembered exactly what I wrote in that email. I felt like a fool – worse, I felt like I was a danger to my friends.

As if the situation wasn't bad enough, I thought back to the day I sent the email. Elle's 30th birthday. Jesus Christ. A few more painful memories flickered through my mind like a demented film reel. The last week of August, Elle added me to her checking account as an authorized user at my behest, getting me my own debit card. Sitting at the Verizon store with her as she tried to get me a new phone and number on her account after I lied to her, once again, that I was done with Aileen and needed to go fully no-contact. The massive dent that spanned the entire side of the car.

And, as the cruel final scene, a memory of sitting on Elle's back porch as a beautiful sunset glowed around us. She told me about big plans she was making for her birthday. The restaurant she dreamed about going to for years. The classy hotel she wanted to stay at for a night after finding a brochure for it at a local rest stop. She carried the brochure around all summer, looking through it when things felt particularly bleak. She asked me if I would like to go with her. Of course I did. Did I mean it at the time, or had I already decided to go back to Aileen and I was just bullshitting her? "Promise? Or are you just saying that and you're going to go back to her and disappear for a month before sending me some absolutely *nasty devastating shit* again?" Was it a serious question, or did she actually trust me and believe me so completely that she was making a joke about our previous dynamic as if it was finally over? And what did I do for her birthday instead? What the hell was wrong with me?

I forced it all out of my mind. I hoped I would be seeing her soon, anyway. My court date in Massachusetts for hitting the guardrail was coming up in less than a week, and maybe she'd be there? It was her car, after all, and she was a passenger. The cops spoke to her that night. I had accidentally given her COVID, and she was so sick at the time that she was finally able to pass out after experiencing near-unbearable kidney pain for hours and didn't even wake up when we hit the guardrail. After I passed every field sobriety test, the cops asked her to finish the rest of the drive home (which she did, gritting her teeth through the pain). Yeah, she'd definitely be there. She had to be.

My court date was on a Tuesday, and I arrived bright and early for my 8:00 a.m. appearance. I pleaded with the Judge, leveraging my mental illness and blaming my unexpected exhaustion on a medication change after being discharged from the hospital. Fortunately, he went for it and took mercy on me. No misdemeanor charge, just a small fine. He even thanked me for making the trip all the way from New York. It was the best possible outcome, except for the fact that Elle wasn't here.

Back at home, a golden opportunity presented itself. I had plans to go out for a beer that night with a new friend, some guy Aileen and I met at a party at a friend's house. His marriage was ending, he needed to get out of the house, whatever. We grabbed a drink at a bar near his place, and I told him we had to make a quick stop before heading to a party. As soon as we were back in the car, I dialed Elle's number.

Somehow, no matter how foul I had been or how long it was since we last spoke, she always picked up when I called. I tried to be funny. "Hey, I'm going out on the town with a friend tonight, and I was calling you to see if you would want to come?"

"YES," she blurted out. "Ahem. Yeah. I'm around, I'm at home. I'll get ready? How long?"

I offered no explanation to the disposable rent-a-friend I was stuck with for the night (he was a cool guy and we definitely had stuff in common, but do you ever get that feeling that someone isn't going to be in your life for long? Yeah.), but he was a guy with a shitty marriage, so he could probably figure out what was going on. I parked the car in the now-familiar parking lot of Elle's apartment. She had been waiting by her front window and came outside when she saw us pull in. Even though I was in a car she hadn't seen before, it was like 10:30 p.m. on a Tuesday night so no one else was coming or going.

I didn't even need to say anything to the new guy; he instantly got a read on the situation and got out to get in the backseat. Elle got in the passenger seat, and I almost couldn't believe we were actually next to each other. My life was so different from the last time we had seen each other. Only two months had passed but it felt like a year. She somehow looked older, more mature? Maybe it was the outfit (black beret, black turtleneck, black bell bottoms, black boots)? Whatever it was, I was into it.

"Oh! Hi," she said to Friend Guy when she noticed him in the backseat. "I'm..." she started to introduce herself but trailed off and shot me a glance. Ah, she wasn't sure if this guy was "safe" or if there was some cover story or fake name she was supposed to have in case word got back to Aileen.

"This is Elle," I jumped in. They exchanged the "nice to meet you" or whatever, and that was basically the last word Friend Guy got in edgewise the entire drive. Elle and I filled every second with conversation and catching up. I could see the gears turning inside her head, a million questions she wanted to ask me, but she was clearly trying hard to make sure she didn't say anything even slightly suspicious. There was so much I wanted to say to her, but it would have been weird with the audience in the backseat.

We spent the night at Niki's apartment. She was getting kicked out of her apartment after squandering her rent money on gambling for so long. She had to be out by the morning and hadn't even started packing yet (typical Niki). Luckily, she knew everyone and plenty of people showed up that night for the moving party. Drinks were being passed around and, knowing Niki's current line of work (hint: it's white and powdery), there was probably more being shared. I made the perfunctory rounds, greeting friends and telling everyone I've been just *great*, thanks for asking. With that out of the way, I pulled Elle into one of the rooms and started packing stuff up.

Within ten minutes, we were laying on our stomachs on the floor, next to each other, in comfortable silence. I should have apologized for the psychotic email, but I didn't. In fact, I usually never apologized or acknowledged prior insanity whenever Elle and I were reunited. She usually didn't press it, at least not this early in the night. We were still just taking in the novelty of being around each other again, and neither of us dared to break that spell.

Despite avoiding the uncomfortable elephant in the room, we somehow found plenty to talk about. Every so often we would join the rest of the party, laugh at whatever YouTube video they put on the TV, and pack up some stuff, before returning to our own little world. After a couple of hours, I realized that I left my phone in the car. I went down to get it and came back upstairs. Without thinking, I turned my phone on to see if any messages had come through.

Fuck. Fuck. Fuck.

The entire reason my phone was off was because Aileen and I had a "safety" tracking app installed on our phones for "accountability". I turned my phone off back at the bar so the app would keep my location there. Now Aileen would see that I was at Niki's apartment in the middle of the night instead of where I told her I would be, and I would have a situation on my hands. I immediately turned my phone off, but the damage was done.

Within minutes, Niki's phone lit up with a venomous text from Aileen, warning her to stay away from me or face consequences. Aileen didn't know there was a party. She thought I was alone. But the silver lining to that (gold, even) was that she also had no idea Elle was there. Fortunately, Niki brushed it off. She was used to threats, and she dealt with far scarier people than Aileen. She took the high road and told Aileen not to worry about it, saying that she'd have done the same thing if she thought her man was alone at some chick's apartment in the middle of the night. Everyone was well aware of Aileen's bullshit and only ever put up with her for my benefit, so I knew no one would out me to her.

After another hour or two of helping Niki pack up her life into boxes, the three of us decided to head out. I dropped off Friend Guy and Elle and I headed back to her apartment. I didn't want her to go just yet, and I could tell she felt the same. We ended up talking for a couple of hours, until the sky turned light gray and we both knew I couldn't plausibly stay any longer. When I got home, Aileen was passed out on the couch.

November was rainy that year and continued in a similar fashion, and I reached out to Elle as often as I could (while being as careful as possible). We were about to lose the car. Even though her dad wasn't making us pay rent, I had so little money coming in (and she wasn't working) that we couldn't afford the car anymore. Both of our driving records were so shot that the insurance was astronomical, too. We were behind a few payments on the car and made a deal with the dealership to just bring it back. I continued trying to rebuild my virtual practice after the chaos of the summer and early fall, but it was still a fraction of the size it was before. I was finally dealing with years' worth of tax returns that needed to be filed and would be on the hook for tens of thousands of dollars, at the very least. This was a massive undertaking and required going through bank statements and receipts for the last several years for deductions.

While living at her dad's house Aileen behaved a little better, but still wasn't making any of the above tasks any easier. She would get mad these things weren't done, then manufacture drama at pivotal moments to keep me from making progress. By the week of Thanksgiving, I was frustrated and sick of it. I uninstalled the tracker app from my phone and reached out to Elle early one morning, telling her that I was on my way in an Uber. We were going to finally take care of my taxes.

When I showed up at her door, she was surprised to see all the stuff I had with me. As always, she was welcoming, and I told her that it was for real this time. I dropped all my stuff off inside her living room then told her that I knew the perfect place to bang out a few years' worth of taxes: the massive library of the college in Southfield. I spent hours and hours studying there while I was in grad school, and I knew it was the perfect place for me to buckle down and focus.

We worked all day and into the night. I told her that I was rebuilding the practice, so whenever my phone would ring with a patient call, I just handed her the phone. She wasn't rusty at all, even though it had been months since she'd last spoken to any patients. As always, we made the perfect team, and after about eighteen hours, we finally had all five years' worth of taxes finished (and not a moment too soon, either, because my appointment at the tax place to hand everything off so they could send it to the IRS was tomorrow).

We crashed on her couch and the next day, Elle and I took everything to Jackson Hewitt for my appointment. I handed everything over and sat there dumbfounded as the preparer told me it would be $400 for everything. Elle excused herself for a moment and called home. After she explained the situation, her ex transferred her the money (have I said yet that Elle and her ex are good people? They're good people). We paid, and I relaxed. Sure, the IRS would process everything and send me a massive bill, but at least I wasn't running from the situation anymore.

Lockwood

The next day was Thanksgiving, and I had asked Nathan to come over to Elle's so we could do some more work to get the practice up and running. He was also helping out by giving Elle one of his old, broken iPhones (I had arrived at Elle's with the cheapest prepaid Android model. She took the SIM card out of her iPhone and lent it to me, leaving her without a phone). I made the usual call to my dad to say I was leaving Aileen for good. Things were humming along!

As the day wore on, though, Aileen started blowing up my phone with texts. Not the usual vitriol, just pictures of the Thanksgiving dishes she had made and questions about when I'd be home for dinner. It started to wear me down, and I told Elle she would need to drive me back to Aileen's for dinner. Given that she had spent three days straight doing free work for me (to say nothing of the emotional component), she was predictably hurt and frustrated. I was a dick.

Things were a blur after this. She was crying, saying her usual sad bullshit: *You said you were leaving her for good. I did everything. It felt so real this time.* Give me a break. As I was putting my shoes on to leave, her ex and Nathan approached me and asked if we could all step outside for a minute. They were telling me that I was never around to see Elle deal with the fallout whenever I did this. it always wrecked her, I needed to stop bouncing between lives based on what was convenient at the time, I was breaking her heart every single time. I realized I was crying. It was incredibly uncomfortable. They were right, but I just wanted it to stop. I said I just needed to divorce Aileen, then I could be with Elle for real.

I went back inside, and Elle was ready to drive me to Aileen's. On the way to her car, she took the cake we bought to celebrate my "new life" and threw it in the road. It wasn't like her to do something so dramatic. Nathan and Elle's ex were right; whenever I did something to hurt her, I was usually so caught up in trying to avoid the fallout from Aileen that I never thought about the impact of my actions.

On the drive to Aileen's father's house, I started crying and I didn't stop. I told Elle that I didn't want this life, this isn't how I wanted to live, it was too much. Once again, I told her how normal and stable my life with Abbie had been. "I know," Elle said. "I've always wanted to give you that."

When we approached Aileen's house, I told Elle to keep driving. She parked at an elementary school at the end of the street. After a few minutes, I told her to take me home. "Aileen's house? Or...?"

"*Home*. My home. Your apartment," I clarified, hoping that I was finally doing the right thing.

The next day was finally the day we agreed to drop the Honda off at the dealership. Seeing it as an opportunity to force me to see her, Aileen started hammering me with texts again. I told her that I did not need to be there for this, and she didn't even need to go inside the dealership at all. Just leave the keys in the car and drop it off. She wasn't hearing it. She finally issued an ultimatum: if I didn't come with her, she wouldn't bring the car back at all. Fine.

I had Elle drop me off at the train station, asking her to stay close to the dealership so she could pick me up afterwards. I told Aileen to come pick me up, giving her a story about how I had gone to Michael's for a few days. She agreed, and we made our way to the dealership.

When we were almost there, Aileen started freaking out. She was screaming at me, and started closed-fist punching me in the head as I was driving. She wouldn't stop, despite the fact that we were on a busy road with four lanes and lots of traffic. I couldn't deal with it anymore and swerved onto a side street to avoid an accident. She wouldn't listen to me and anything I said just made her punch harder. Out of options, I jumped out of the car and took off on foot. I ran the wrong way up one-way streets, hoping she wouldn't follow.

I ran until I was out of breath, looking over my shoulder the entire time. Eventually, I had to stop to catch my breath. I crouched behind a fast food restaurant and called Elle to come get me. I was sobbing and panicking, but somehow, she understood what I was saying. I told her where I was, and she came to get me. She handed me her scarf to blow my nose with, and eventually, I calmed down a little.

By the time we got back to Elle's parking lot, Aileen started texting me her usual "come back" sob story, and I engaged. Elle kept asking if I was ready to go inside yet, and I showed her my phone and said I was almost done. "What the fuck?" Elle said after looking at the screen. "You guys are just like, insulting me?"

"Don't worry about it, I'm just messing with her head," I said, completely unconvincingly. At that point, I had made up my mind, and I didn't really care *what* Elle believed. It was almost midnight, but I told Elle that I needed to make a private phone call to my father and asked her to drive me fifteen minutes away to the 24-hour CVS in Bergen. It was extremely unconvincing, but I could tell she bought it.

When she parked at CVS, I looked her straight in the eye and said, in the nastiest tone I could summon, "There is no *'us'*." I hopped out of the car and walked around the side of the CVS and called Aileen. Eventually, Elle got out of her car and came over, crying. She started to say something, but I cut her off, loud enough for Aileen to hear: "You were our admin, a long time ago. But I'm a happily married man. You must have hallucinated and read into things. I'm a happily married man." I was delusional at best.

I kept repeating that over and over, getting louder any time she tried to talk. I caught snippets of what she was saying – the $400 I owed her ex for the tax stuff, everything I left at her apartment, how I was still using her phone. Not my problem. I repeated everything over and over until she finally got fed up and left. After she was gone, Aileen told me that her father could come bring her to get me, but not for a couple of hours. I called a friend, who picked me up without asking too many questions. We hung out in his garage as he dressed a deer he had recently killed. We had venison back strap that night.

Eventually, Aileen and her father arrived to come get me. Aileen didn't punish me too much (I guess she got it all out of her system when she beat me up earlier that day), and her father said he was just happy that I was okay. For some reason, I thought I was happy, too. In reality, I was just going back into the lion's den. The next morning, Elle called to ask about getting her iPhone back. I pretended I had no idea what she was referring to and handed the phone to Aileen, who took the opportunity to bellow "Elle, you're not pretty!" into the microphone. She handed the phone back to me, and I saw that Elle had hung up.

People always ask why I went back. They imagine it's weakness, or that I must have liked the pain. The truth is uglier. Abuse rewires you. You start living for the rare moments of kindness like a gambler chasing one more win, convincing yourself the good times are proof the nightmare can end. Every insult, every betrayal, is followed by just enough love to keep you hooked. They tear you down until you forget what whole feels like, then convince you they're the only one who can fix you. I didn't go back because I loved her, I went back because she made me believe I couldn't live without her.

In the coming days, I realized that returning to Aileen's had been a mistake. Things got so bad that I attempted suicide, again, this time with a massive dose of Klonopin. Her father was actually the one to call 911; Aileen probably would have left me in the basement indefinitely. By the time I was released from the hospital, I knew that something needed to change. I may have been sober, but I needed a break to work on myself.

I got on a plane in late December 2022, headed to Florida for a 30-day dual-diagnosis inpatient rehab program. The program at River Oaks was robust without being over-the-top, and basically everyone on staff there had run into addiction at one point in their lives. A few of the therapists there had even spent time in Gladiator School (which I understand now, even though it didn't mean much to me at the time). This place was the real deal.

I spent the entire thirty days working on myself, with no Aileen around to fuck things up whenever I achieved some semblance of peace or balance. I could see others around me squandering their time in the program, torpedoing their chances at sobriety by bringing in drugs, trying to sneak in a few hookups, or getting into fights. Years ago, that was me, at Silver Hill with my rehab girlfriend. Not this time.

I arrived home a month later, with a clear head and a new perspective. I was ready to do things right this time, vowing to take my relationship with Aileen seriously and give it one more real chance. When you're away from someone for thirty days, it's easy to convince yourself that they're not the problem. She was traumatized, she lost her kids, maybe I had been the "bad spouse" all along. Again, I desperately didn't want to fail another marriage, and blaming everything on myself made me feel like at least I was in control of the situation.

Fortunately, Aileen had gotten a job at a salon while I was at River Oaks. I secured an office at a local coworking space and started rebuilding my practice for the millionth time. I secretly reached out to Elle, asking if she knew a site where I could commission a new logo for the practice. She was thrilled to hear from me, and said those sites were a rip-off and she could make one for me herself.

I paid her $50 for the logo and coordinating business cards, and $50 to design a website. Everything looked flawless and professional, and she admitted that she taught herself how to use Photoshop in order to make this stuff for me. I was enthralled with the stuff she made, but I started to feel guilty and wanted to make sure everyone was on the same page. I called her and made sure she knew that I had made up my mind, and I would be spending the rest of my domestic life with Aileen. I could tell she wasn't thrilled, but she understood, and wanted to make sure I knew that she wasn't doing this stuff for that reason.

I really did try my hardest with Aileen, but it was clear to me that there was nothing between us. The relationship was hollow. Her job stabilized her a little bit, as did her father's presence. But our relationship was built on chaos, so the calmness only amplified the lack of true connection we had. Every time I tried to actually *talk* with her, I was shocked at how shallow she truly was. I guess when you're on drugs all the time and dealing with a never-ending stream of crises, you never have a chance to realize that you've never actually had a real, fulfilling conversation with the other person.

We went through the motions, working, going to couples counseling as requested by CPS, making weekly visits to Lorenzo at my parents' house. Even my parents could see how depressed and anxious I was. My mom pulled me aside during one of the visits to ask, "When are you finally going to leave this girl?" It was that obvious. At home, I spent as much time as possible stoned on medical marijuana and watching Netflix so we wouldn't have to talk.

By that point, I was paying Elle $50 a week to answer the phones, and we ramped up marketing until I had a full practice again. She respected what I said about Aileen, and stayed professional. But by late spring, my feelings had become so strong that I couldn't ignore them anymore. Elle was sitting on the floor of my office at the coworking space, putting together a bookshelf. Trying to sound nonchalant to hide the burning desire I was actually feeling, I poked her on the shoulder. "Hey, when you're done with that, do you think it would be okay if I kissed you?"

She smiled.

The Exit Wound

I spent the summer getting my affairs in order. I started slowly moving my things into Elle's house, stuff Aileen wouldn't notice was missing. I had a separation agreement drawn up. I finally got myself a vehicle, too. The interest was insane because of my credit, and I had to put down a massive down payment, but it was mine (Aileen made it clear many times over that the Nissan was hers, even though I made all the payments, and threatened to call the police to report it stolen any time I attempted to go for a drive after we fought). She knew things were dying, and when she saw my new car, the only thing she had to say was that now I was going to leave her.

On September 9, 2023, I confirmed Aileen's suspicions and left her. Her father was out of the house, and she used the opportunity to start a bullshit fight. After the fight, she went for a walk, and I knew I had my chance. I got in my car and drove through the neighborhood until I found her at the elementary school at the end of the street. I don't know what she expected, but it definitely wasn't me presenting the separation agreement to her. In the agreement, I offered several large lump-sum payments to her in lieu of alimony. She was offended that I thought she would accept being "paid off" to leave the marriage. Of course, her offense evaporated when I offered more money. She agreed to the terms, and I texted Elle that I finally did it and I was on my way to her apartment.

Despite how bad things had been, it still took all of my courage and sober energy to leave. Breaking away from a sociopath is much harder than it looks. But with everything said and done, I'd rather go to federal prison than spend another minute of my life as a slave to someone as hollow and cold as her.

Life post-sociopath still had its difficulties. Aileen had agreed to the separation thinking that it was temporary and I would soon "come to my senses" and return to her, and I had to lean into that to convince her to get the documents notarized so the separation would be official. At Elle's house, I had vivid nightmares for months, unable to get more than a couple hours of rest without waking up in a sweat. On my third night after leaving Aileen, I emptied the entire contents of my bowels in bed while sleeping, like my body was finally releasing all the toxicity from the poisonous relationship.

Adderall and Other False Prophets

I suffered random panic attacks in the weeks after the split, leaving me paralyzed and unable to travel or do anything fun. It was like a toxin was leaving my body, and it wasn't going to go quietly. Any communication I had with Aileen seemed to re-trigger the "toxic" effect, and I tried to limit any interaction with her to only the most necessary aspects of the pending divorce. Any time I saw her or spoke to her, I felt sick for days.

I mentioned this to my father on a visit to see Lorenzo. He told me that something similar was happening to the child as well. Whenever Aileen would make a rare visit to see Lorenzo, he would have nightmares and behavioral changes for several days afterwards. He noted this pattern and had already turned it over to Lorenzo's therapists and CPS.

After we got everything notarized and I handed off the first series of checks to her as specified in the agreement, I was able to avoid contact with Aileen. The effect this had on me was incredible. I still had issues of my own to deal with, but life without Aileen was much more peaceful. It wasn't until I was gone that I realized that it didn't matter how hard I tried or what I did, as long as we were together, I had no chance at a thriving, happy, healthy life.

Once upon a time, I read a book on sociopaths. The book had very clear recommendations on how to deal with them: run away, as fast as you can. You will not beat them; if you have any emotional tone whatsoever, the sociopath already has the advantage. Don't get angry or attempt to mudsling, because they'll return it a hundred times worse. Ignore them, get out, and start over from nothing if you have to. And that's what I ended up doing. I left a lot behind the day I took off (like a $22,000.00 diamond ring, a $17,000.00 Persian rug, and a $4,000.00 mattress, for starters). But stuff can be replaced; your sanity and years of your life cannot. Despite the high dollar amounts, it wasn't worth it to me to try and recover those items. If it meant I would have to speak to her even once more than necessary, the price was too high (no pun intended).

With things calm and no immediate crisis looming for the first time in years, it felt like I could finally focus on moving forward. It had been a while since I'd spoken to Jason Hendrix about the one million shares of preferred stock I held and the acquisition of Synaptic Link Telehealth (which had been renamed

PrimeMed shortly before it was sold for around $30 million to a much larger telehealth company). The problem was, I had no clue where my shares were, or what they were now worth.

That's where Warren came in. He was a good friend and a brilliant attorney, already a partner at a massive firm before hitting forty. Warren and I went way back. Ours was one of those rare friendships built on trust, mutual respect, and a long history. I still remember when Warren invited me to his office and gave me a full tour like it was his home. The place was overwhelming. I couldn't wrap my head around the idea of hundreds of lawyers all packed into one building, debating issues on behalf of the firm. I made plans with him to meet up and discuss the shares.

At his office, he sat me down and had someone bring me a coffee (he and I were still caffeine junkies) and we started talking. I filled him in on the issues I was juggling, including dealing with the SCR (as soon as CPS found out Aileen and I were separated, my case with family court evaporated. However, by that point, the wheels had been in motion so long that New York had placed me on the parental abuse and neglect registry. Aileen was found guilty of neglecting her kids, and even though we weren't yet married when the offense occurred, we were married when they put her on the registry, so they included me as well) and trying to track down and litigate for my corporate shares. Apparently, when the acquisition went through, my shares were transferred to the acquiring company. Warren and his team were able to see that in real time.

They couldn't determine the exact value of the shares, but estimated they were worth somewhere between $500,000 and $1.5 million. His firm was more than willing to litigate to recover them, but even at a discounted rate, the price tag was around $30,000 up front (and that was only for the shares. Appealing the decision to put me on the SCR would be separate). At that point, I didn't have that kind of liquid cash, though I figured I could start saving and maybe ask my father for help. Warren reassured me that the shares would remain available to pursue until January 2025. I had over a year. Plenty of time.

I went to my father thinking this would be easy (it was a sure thing, and I'd pay him back from the proceeds) but he wanted nothing to do with it. Ouch. So I started saving the money myself, knowing I could pull it together in six months, no problem. Finally, after living through so much chaotic insanity, maybe I'd actually be rewarded. I had given up my family, my life, basically everything. Now, with money, I could make it up to everyone. At the very least, the kids would have college funds, private school, brand-name clothes, you name it.

I knew that I could get $30,000 no problem. The practice was doing great, and I was also in the midst of opening a concierge mobile IV wellness service. There were plenty of IV wellness places locally, but we'd be the first to bring the mobile concierge model from the big cities to Upstate New York. I had the LLC set up, all the supplies purchased, and the website, logo, and marketing materials that Elle designed looked just as good as the stuff coming out of LA and NYC. I was just about to hire an RN to set the lines. The margins on wellness IVs were insane; it would be like printing money once we opened for business.

All I had to do was stay out of trouble and not become a criminal in the meantime. Life would be golden. Piece of cake. With two income streams, I could pay Warren's retainer in no time. I shut out everything else in my life and focused singularly on making the money.

Elle and I were working full-time hours for the practice, then putting in full-time hours making preparations for the IV business. The only time I let loose was during our weekly trips to the VR every Friday. She was sick of going every week, and looking back, she had some good points. She was tired of working nonstop all week, dealing with my moods and volatility and completing the endless tasks I thanklessly gave her, only to see me being fun and talkative and social with the strippers, who hadn't "earned" my kindness like she had. Since she was helping with the IV stuff, I paid her $100 a week, but she was annoyed that I would have no problem blowing twice (or even three times) that much on one girl at the club.

She was also annoyed at how much I talked about the RN I was planning to hire for the IV business. This was a fair assessment; I was constantly commenting on how much I enjoyed talking to her. I told Elle that I would have to pay the RN $50 an hour, but she understood, right? I had to be competitive if I wanted the best employees. And in my mind, this nurse was the best. Sure, Elle may have found evidence of questionable decision-making (she had posted TikTok videos from her hospital job with patients in the background), but I was the boss and I knew what I was doing.

I ignored every concern Elle brought to me, writing it off as jealousy. She withdrew, but I was able to ignore it as long as she was getting the work done. At 11:00 a.m. on Christmas, I dragged her back to the office as soon as Siobhan had opened her last present. I started to get stressed out, wondering how I would ever get the new business off the ground without Adderall or cocaine to keep me going. With my brain fried from nitrous and ever-increasing doses of Klonopin, I became mean. We started to fight, and she was sick of my shit.

My last family court date was January 8, 2024. Seeing Aileen had thrown me into a tailspin, and I took it out on Elle. She finally decided to stand up for herself, and told me that she wasn't breaking up with me or kicking me out, but if I was going to keep acting like this, she would go sleep in the hallway. This sent me into an immediate rage, and I got nasty, insulting her apartment and telling her I would be more than happy to move back in with Aileen and employ her instead. I whipped my vape at her, hitting her in the head. I do not handle drugs well.

Her ex, our roommate, heard the commotion and came into our room. This was the first time I'd seen him anything but calm, and we started fighting. I wasn't thinking, only reacting to perceived threats. I pushed him to the ground, and Elle convinced both of us that everything was fine and to break it up. I saw the massive lump on Elle's head and immediately came back to reality. As her ex left the room, I caught a glimpse in the hallway of Siobhan, who heard everything.

Right away, I was overcome with guilt. I was balled up on the floor, sobbing, while Elle tried to comfort me. I couldn't believe how badly I fucked up, again. We talked, and I promised to do better from that point forward.

The next morning, January 9, 2024, I was arrested. My world collapsed. Everything was gone in an instant.

Aileen had been submitting false reports about me to the DEA since 2022, even during points of our relationship that were "good". No, I wasn't an international drug smuggler or dealer like she claimed. But that didn't seem to matter. She lied under affidavit, but no one cared. She was just a disposable, delusional source. The final nail in the coffin was a pissed-off family member of

Jessica's, hoping to get back at her by making a report to the DEA. I was just caught in the crossfire and, even though I was later able to produce a text message from the person who made the report proving that they lied, it didn't matter.

The damage was done. That day, I stopped being a provider and became a defendant. I met with the Judge before being thrown in county jail to get my head straight. I had been taking a lot of Klonopin, and the Judge was aware of it. He wanted me clear-headed, to actually grasp what was happening. At the time, I wasn't even close to processing the severity of it all.

Those days in solitary were terrifying. I had no idea what was happening, and prison had always been my biggest fear. I drifted in and out of sleep, staring at the blue bars and the COs pacing outside, watching the inmates. There was no way out. No one filled me in on what exactly was going on, so I didn't know if this was going to be my forever or just a temporary stop. I was in an orange jumpsuit and plastic clogs, caught in a haze of confusion.

A guy came by three times a day with boxed meals, trying to get me to eat, but my body was in shock (it still is, in some ways). I was stuck in survival mode, and food felt like an alien concept. My sweat soaked into the jumpsuit. By the third day, I must have reeked. Strangely enough, my hair was still perfectly combed, the pomade keeping it in the exact same shape as when I left the apartment on Tuesday morning.

Relief came only in my dreams. I saw Elle, Abbie, my family, the ocean. My brain was working overtime to confabulate an acceptable reality. But every time I woke up, I was still in that same cold box, alone, staring at the guards, the blue bars, and the untouched stack of food beside me.

I remember being brought in shackles to a closed room with a partition, unable to see who was on the other side. That's where I was first introduced to the public defender I had been assigned. He was just a disembodied voice, asking me a series of questions while I stood there.

He told me I'd likely be released on probation while awaiting trial, and that it should happen the next time I saw the Judge. I wasn't even sure how long I'd been in here or what day it was. Through our conversation, I was able to ascertain that it was now Wednesday, I had been arrested the day before, and I'd be back in court to see the Judge tomorrow. Still in shock, this information meant nothing to me. I heard what he was saying, but my brain wasn't processing any of it. Afterward, they brought me back to my cell. I laid down and tried to fall asleep, hoping to see familiar faces or at least some beautiful landscape in my dreams.

Thursday came, and a CO woke me up to tell me I had court that day. I was going to be transported with other prisoners to the courthouse downtown. I refused breakfast again, but I could tell by the food they offered that it was morning. They shackled me up and brought me out of my cell, down a series of hallways, and into a holding room with other inmates. I tried hard not to make eye contact with anyone. I didn't want to invite trouble.

At one point, two prisoners got into it. Evidently one had some beef with the other, and they started grappling, trying to force each other to the floor. The COs didn't respond until the noise got too loud and there was blood everywhere. When they finally came in, they did it in full riot gear. Everyone hit the floor with their hands laced behind their heads, and I followed suit. The two guys who had fought were removed, and the rest of us were loaded into a transport vehicle, all chained together like a chain gang.

The ride to the courthouse was disorienting. We couldn't see the street, but I could tell it was a sunny, cold day with a bit of wind. Once we arrived, we were unloaded and brought into holding cells in the basement of the courthouse. I ended up paired with a guy who wasn't too bad. He told me he was Mohican, and that he was in for shielding his mother from a charge. I remember thinking the bathroom in that cell was a massive upgrade compared to the one I had in solitary. Eventually, a courthouse CO came through and handed out lunch to everyone in a brown paper bag. My stomach still in knots, I passed my lunch off to my cellmate.

I don't remember being led out of my cell when it was my turn with the Judge. Suddenly, I was standing in the courtroom, listening to the prosecutor say I was "facing 25 to life" in prison. Holy fucking shit – what was happening? I couldn't do life in prison. That just wasn't going to work for me. This couldn't be real life.

The Judge decided to release me on probation, but at the time I had no idea what that even meant. I remember being told to leave the courtroom after the Judge finished, and when I turned around, I was stunned to see Elle there. She looked exhausted and teary-eyed, but I was so relieved to see a familiar face. I caught her eye and smiled, lifting up my hands to show her the cuffs and shrugging. My last memory of the courtroom was her smiling back at me before the COs whisked me away, back to the holding cell to wait while the rest of the prisoners had their turn in front of the Judge.

On the way back to the jail, I was seated at the very front of the cattle car. I could see the backs of the COs, one driving and one in the passenger seat. They both had their phones out, with one playing a porn video and the other casually scrolling through photos of kilos of marijuana. It was a moment of unexpected comedy for me and the guys who could see through the little window into the truck's cabin.

We got back late and missed dinner, but I didn't care. As we re-entered the jail, I told the guards that the Judge said I was to be released. They heard me but still threw me back in my solitary cell. I was confused and scared, wondering if maybe I'd misheard the Judge – maybe I wasn't getting out after all, and I'd be stuck here indefinitely awaiting trial. Why did it seem like nobody was on the same page, and why couldn't I get a straight answer out of anyone?

Back in my cell, I realized I had a new neighbor, a transgender woman. She was talking with the guards about a rumor she'd heard earlier. Supposedly, some new prisoner had smuggled in a large stash of crack cocaine in their colon. I remember wondering what exactly the smuggler planned to do with it once they got it into the jail. We were under constant supervision, so smoking it or trying to find a hiding spot for it would be impossible. Still, it was a ridiculous story, and for a moment, it distracted me.

After entertaining the guards with her story, my neighbor turned her attention to me and started making small talk. She was the kindest person I'd met in three days, and while I was grateful for the company, it wasn't enough to keep me out of my own head for long. Time dragged on, and whatever hope I had of being released started to fade. But then, around 9:00 p.m., the guards came to my cell and told me I was being let out. I was ecstatic. I wished my new neighbor good luck, changed back into my clothes, and went to the front desk to ask them to call Elle so she could come pick me up.

Lockwood

For the first time since I'd met her, Elle didn't answer my call. That's when I realized that her phone must have been taken by the DEA as evidence since it was physically inside the office when they did their raid. The only other number I knew by heart was my parents' landline back home.

They didn't make the release easy. I wasn't allowed to wait inside the jail for a cab, so on the night of January 11, 2024, I stepped out into the freezing dark wearing nothing but a sports jacket, jeans, and dress shoes. I started walking, and soon a state trooper drove by. He slowed down, lowered his window, and looked me over before commenting, "Nice jacket." I wanted to ask him for a ride but was too afraid he'd bring me back to the jail. Instead, I kept walking that pitch-black road away from the jail, chasing the faint promise of light until the main road finally came into view.

There was a gas station right on the corner, and I practically threw myself against the door. The attendant was kind, despite how crazy and beat-up I must have looked. I was hyperventilating and half-frozen, and he let me drink as much hot coffee as I needed. After I had warmed up a little bit, I asked him if I could use a phone to call my dad. He agreed, and I wondered if he was used to people in my situation. My dad called me a cab, and I thanked the gas station attendant for everything he did for me that night.

The cab pulled up, and I had never been so relieved to get a ride in my life. The driver asked me what was going on, and I told him. I saw him take a long drag off a cigarette, and I suddenly snapped to attention. With everything else going on, I hadn't even realized that I was in nicotine withdrawal, but now it was all I could think about. I asked him for the butt end of his cigarette, and he passed it back to me. That first drag of nicotine was better than anything I'd ever tasted.

When I got back to Elle's apartment, I was relieved to see the lights were on and the door was unlocked. I came inside and quietly called out *Hello?*

"OH MY FUCKING GOD," she cried, flying around the corner to the entryway where I stood. I collapsed into her arms, tears in my eyes, still in full-blown shock. She held me and told me she had been at the prison all day waiting for me, but they hadn't released me until much later than expected. Just like I thought, they had taken her phone. Her ex was tied up in traffic court that night, and when the inmate notification system told her I'd been released, she emailed Nathan and asked him to call the jail so they could tell me she was on her way. They told Nathan I would be waiting in the lobby, and Elle jumped in the car with Siobhan. When she arrived, they gave her the runaround and said there must have been some miscommunication because I left already. They wouldn't tell her if I left on foot or got picked up, so she drove around for a bit looking for me. Unsuccessful, she finally returned home about a half hour before I got there.

I couldn't believe I was finally back home with Elle. It almost didn't feel real. I tried to explain what was going on, but I still wasn't even fully sure. All I knew was that I had to report for probation in the morning, something I'd never done before. Just another terrifying step into the unknown. The Judge had also instructed me to retain private counsel, so I already knew where the $20,000 sitting in my checking account was going. I paced the apartment, muttering to myself, still not eating or drinking (it took weeks and a weight loss of forty-five pounds before I could eat normally again). I was completely shell-shocked. That first night, I couldn't sleep. Elle and I sat on the couch watching reruns, just trying to fill the silence with something.

Early the next morning, I got up with Elle and headed back to the courthouse for my first probation meeting. I was scared shitless. The whole way there, I kept thinking they were going to throw me back in jail. I didn't understand the process. None of it made sense. She did her best to reassure me, and soon we were sitting side-by-side in the cold, uncomfortable waiting area of the federal probation office.

I met Nick, my probation officer. He was a man in his forties, with a full sleeve of tattoos down his right arm and a surprisingly empathetic demeanor for someone who clearly didn't take any nonsense. At my initial visit, he took my photo and walked me through what was essentially an intake interview, asking a series of questions meant to get a sense of who I was, what meds I was on, and what kind of environment I lived in.

Then it was time for a urine drug screen. I tested positive for THC for a while, which made sense since I had a medical card and used it at night to help me sleep. Nick understood that it was legal in New York and I had a medical card, but

I had to follow federal rules now (as in, weed was still completely federally illegal, so I had to quit or else I'd be violating the terms of probation). I had to call a number every night to find out whether I had to come in for a drug test the next day, and they were completely random. At first, I got called in once a week. After a year of clean tests, they called me in less than once a month.

He also let me know he'd be conducting a house visit soon, so Elle and I made sure to clear out anything questionable – weed, paraphernalia, all of it went straight into the trash. When he came by to inspect the apartment, everything went smoothly. We passed.

As part of the terms of my probation, I could no longer prescribe controlled substances. That meant no more Klonopin for me, which was almost as scary as everything else that had happened. Discontinuing a drug like Klonopin requires medical supervision, which I didn't have. In jail, they gave me the smallest dose possible to keep me from having seizures, but I was on my own after that. The supply I'd been taking came from a friend (something I obviously never should have done) and now I was left to deal with withdrawal on my own. I was navigating Klonopin withdrawal, psychological shock, and basic survival (trying to eat, drink, sleep) all at once.

I was in a dangerous place, but I pushed through. I had a prescription for Gabapentin and used it to manage the taper, though I barely had enough. A withdrawal of that magnitude typically requires 45 to 60 days of coverage, and I was working with far less. I counted out every pill and built a schedule that kept me just this side of a seizure. I couldn't sleep. I couldn't eat. I just paced the house, hour after hour, waiting to see if I'd fall apart. The Gabapentin held me together by a thread. It was brutal, and I wouldn't wish it on anyone (except maybe Aileen).

The beginning of probation was very tough. Shock, withdrawal, weight loss, insomnia. Pacing and pacing and pacing. I still wasn't eating, barely drinking. My body was trying to shut down, but I wouldn't let it. I fought tooth and nail, day after day, night after night. Eventually, I slowly started eating again. I made an appointment with a psychiatrist and a GP. They gradually adjusted the ten medications I was on, and I eventually managed to move from critical to somewhat stable. As long as my life had structure and purpose, I started to feel like things were okay. But letting go of what I loved, being a psych NP, was one of the hardest things I've ever done. That job had been a dream realized through years of hard work, and I lost it for the worst possible reasons: Aileen, drugs, and compromised mental health.

If I could ever start over, I don't know if I'd prescribe controlled substances again. The DEA doesn't care about non-controlled meds. No one warned me to be cautious about what I was prescribing or how much. That kind of heads-up would've been nice. The DEA could see exactly what was being prescribed. They watched me for years, saw the same prescribing patterns, saw the mistakes, and said nothing. If they really thought I was making dangerous decisions, why did they wait so long? They waited until I'd written just enough scripts to justify moving in and making an arrest. They never stepped in, never tried to correct me. They just let the rope run out long enough to make sure it would hang me.

Even though I had cleaned up quite a bit since my lowest point, I was still a tasty case for the DEA. The new chief investigative officer needed something to do, and unfortunately, that something was me. It quickly became clear that this case wasn't what they expected (no one got hurt, no one was selling drugs, and I didn't profit a single cent from what they were accusing me of), but they weren't going to let it go.

So what did the DEA do? They arrested me over Jessica's prescriptions, then dug through the prescribing history of all my patients, looking for anything else they considered criminal. They ended up cherry-picking a handful of patients and claimed that every controlled medication those patients received had been diverted, usually because my notes for those patients weren't current. That was enough for them to slap me with a jail sentence.

On January 9th, they raided the apartment before coming to the office. Fortunately, Siobhan was at school, but Elle's ex wasn't so lucky. He worked from home, so he opened the door to a swarm of DEA officers. They put him in handcuffs while they tore the place apart in an ultimately-unsuccessful search for drugs. He'd later tell us that the most dramatic 'find' of the day was a magazine full of ammo on the living room couch...until one of the officers sheepishly admitted it was his and hadn't been secured properly. The DEA clearly hadn't sent their A-team.

This was even more evident by the time they got to the office. Elle and I were completely unaware of what was going on, but we both had the same panicked idea: ditch any prescriptions we had on us, legitimate or not. Despite being handcuffed and under close watch while the officers raided the office and bagged up everything for evidence, Elle was able to ditch a prescription bottle of Abilify in the compartment of an upholstered chair where the cushion came off for storage. An agent came and sat down on that chair for twenty minutes, complaining about how uncomfortable his bulletproof vest was. They never found it (but they did need an expert to confirm that the bottle of Advil they found in my car was actually Advil, so...yeah).

As for me? I managed to ditch my bottle of Zoloft while under direct surveillance by two DEA agents at their headquarters, with at least six cameras watching me. I had a feeling they were going to want the Zoloft and Abilify. Somehow, they missed both. That alone shows you how green this team was. And maybe it was something else, not antidepressants – my memory is a bit fuzzy (it was an incredibly chaotic day, after all).

I'm sure I'd been on the DEA's radar for years. I was a flagrant drug addict, and they probably knew it. But they also knew I was destroying myself, not anyone else. Maybe that's why there wasn't a single senior agent on my legal case. I even have an FBI number now, even though they were completely disinterested in me. Still, I was issued my very own serial number, like some twisted rite of passage.

My sentencing date got pushed back over and over again, and my attorney came right out and told me that the court has more pressing matters than my case. I don't disagree, but it still sucks to be on their leash, stuck in purgatory until they decide they have time to choose my fate. Meanwhile, real criminals like Aileen keep trudging along, abusing drugs, kids, family, anyone unlucky enough to cross her path. The worst part? I learned the hard way that the first person to call the cops usually wins. Whoever makes the report first turns the other person into the defendant. Aileen was a master of that game. And since she'd apparently been feeding the DEA information since at least 2022, she beat me to the phone.

Adderall and Other False Prophets

At least since my arrest in January 2024, I've reconnected with my family, my friends, and, most importantly, my sons. If I hadn't been arrested, I probably would still be out there chasing the holy grail of success, blind to the fact that my relationships with the people I love had nearly vanished. If nothing else, I was able to finally see things from a new perspective. I've come to understand what actually matters, and what never did.

Charmed and Chained: My Infernal Affair

I've spent a lot of time talking about how destructive Aileen was and the pain she inflicted on those around her. But I hung around for years. I can blame it on my drug addiction, but that isn't the full story. The truth is, despite everything, I really thought I was in love with her. I was even able to convince myself that she loved me, too. I thought that our problems were temporary, that the toxicity was just her impulsive reactions to my own failings. As embarrassing as it is to admit, I tried more than once to salvage the relationship, imagining I could mold her into some version of the perfect housewife like the one I saw in my own upbringing. Not that I should ever compare her to my mother; Aileen could barely manage her chickens without screwing it up. What I really wanted was the full picture: house, wife, kids, and total control. I didn't want to feel vulnerable or lost. I craved the kind of stability and confidence I imagined would make me whole. When Giovanni was born, something shifted. I felt pushed aside by Abbie, like I wasn't needed anymore – or worse, like I didn't even deserve to be around. No this was not the case but I thought it at that time. I wasn't fit to be a father. I was too broken, too far gone. I obsessed over that feeling, chasing answers wherever I could find them. I just didn't know how far that search would take me.

My home life with Abbie and Giovanni started to represent failure to me, so I pulled as far away from it as possible. My entire identity became my clinical work, the telehealth company, and Adderall, a combination that appealed to both the giving and selfish parts of myself. With Adderall, I felt confident, focused, and emotionally dulled – able to push harder and get more done. It became my first real love, filling the void at a time where I didn't feel wanted or in control. At first, I was prescribed it legitimately, but I quickly needed more to achieve the same effect. I stopped going home after work and would stay out late, either building the business or surrounding myself with shady people who enabled and facilitated my new addiction. I told myself I was investing in my child's future, that the hours and effort was for him. But in truth, this was just a lie I leaned on to avoid going home to a wife who loved me and a newborn son she was raising on her own.

Adderall and Other False Prophets

I rode the Adderall train for a while, working eighteen-hour days without sleep, often just changing my shirt so the staff would think I'd gone home. I was in a state of hypomania, and for a time, it worked. I kept that schedule going longer than anyone should. Eventually, though, I had to tap out. That's when I checked into Silver Hill. I told myself I just needed a break, and that once I got out, I could go right back to the grind. But I came back in worse shape than when I went in, hollow and desperate for something more than Adderall and work. I was still too scared to look fear in the eyes and understand the deeper meaning behind what I was feeling. As all of these factors converged, the perfect storm began to form. And that's when I met Aileen – February 21, 2017, working her shift at the strip club.

As evil as she would end up being, *I* was ultimately the one who chose to find meaning in a relationship with someone I normally wouldn't have spoken to beyond a passing hello. I think that was the main reason she was able to get so close to me without raising alarms – I never saw her as someone I'd date. Just a broke stripper, likely stuck in an abusive relationship, and unlike anyone I'd ever been around. I thought I had the upper hand and could run circles around her mentally. I had a master's degree and worked in psych, so I assumed I'd always be able to spot any potential manipulation a mile away. I was in danger and didn't even know it.

Still, there were things about her I found attractive. She possessed qualities I didn't see in my relationship with Abbie, at least not from where I stood at the time. When I met Aileen, I immediately felt a sense of control. She deferred to me on everything – intelligence, life decisions, the big picture. I was the expert, and we talked for hours that night. For once, it felt good to be the one with the upper hand. Abbie was much smarter than me and, as a result, I had always felt a little inferior. But talking to Aileen boosted my confidence, and this enabled her to gain my trust quickly. She knew exactly what she was doing. She came from a world where men go to feel better about themselves, not worse. I was the archetypal strip club patron, marriage falling apart, addiction just taking hold. Her home life was just as wrecked, and she was actively looking for someone new. We were both on the same page and, even though we had just met, it felt natural to spend the night in my hotel room, doing drugs and having sex for the first time.

The sex was pretty good, elevating me to a new level (especially combined with the preexisting highs of cocaine, Adderall, and my position of authority as an NP running a huge practice). She was feeding my confidence, paving over my pain with drugs, sex, and the sense that I was fully in-control. She mirrored my emotional tone, which was reserved, and that felt reassuring. I didn't feel vulnerable, and Aileen was a great distraction from everything unraveling in my life. She saved me from having to process the collapse of my relationship with Abbie and Giovanni. Suddenly, I felt confident in myself and my decisions, and I kept Aileen close. I mistakenly saw her as this newfound "positive" influence in my life, and I didn't want to lose her.

Still, I didn't tell my colleagues or staff about her. Why did I feel the need to hide her? Some part of me remained rational enough to recognize that this probably wasn't a wise decision. I knew that those I respected wouldn't understand what I saw in her. Vlad said at one point, "She's a black widow who will consume you." Abbie said, "She's dark, Asher. There's an energy to her that scares me." Everyone around me saw her for what she was – a sociopath – but I had a completely different take. I saw what I wanted to see. In my hypomanic state, I convinced myself I could mold her and her three children into the perfect family. We'd be normal, happy. I would be in control at all times. I'd learn how to run a family and be a dad, "practicing" on Aileen and her children, so I could someday reenter Abbie's life as an accomplished man.

The fighting and toxicity started gradually, but I got used to it quickly. The pain she inflicted on me started to feel acceptable and even deserved because of what I had done to Abbie and Giovanni. Over time, Aileen slowly evolved from the person who had initially attracted me into someone far more diabolical and calculated. Still, I stayed. Despite her behavior and the undeniable amount of damage she had inflicted (both physical and emotional), I found a warped sense of comfort in how familiar our dynamic had become. I also didn't want to fail another marriage, so I convinced myself to stick it out, again and again. I had already lost so much, and the thought of losing Aileen as well felt like too much to bear. But ultimately, through sobriety and strong support, I finally accepted that she was keeping me isolated and empty by design. It became clear: I had to get out. And so, I did.

"Here in the darkness, I know myself. Can't break free until I let it go. Let me go..." -Amy Lee. Probably one of my favorite lyrics ever. Amy really bottom-lines the choice that must be made in any situation involving mental illness, addiction, abuse, or any other tough situation. I came to see and understand myself as dark and evil, which made it easier to justify terrible behavior and drug abuse. I had so many mental "outs," an endless list of excuses that allowed me to keep going down the dark roads I was on. There was safety in that version of me because I didn't have to feel anything, and the drugs did a phenomenal job at keeping emotions out of reach. If everyone (me included) always expected me to fuck up, I'd never have to feel like people were disappointed in me.

There in the darkness, I knew a version of myself that thrived. But I wouldn't break free until I let the darkness go. I had to commit to sanity and walk away from the sanctuary of drug addiction and an abusive relationship. Identifying as a victim of domestic violence only further justified my drug use. My mania was fueled by cocaine and Adderall, which fed into illusions of grandeur and gave me the energy to live in that delusion. While others around me partook in the darkness too, I believed that my reasons were somehow more justifiable or "correct". Meanwhile, my sons were growing up without me. Every now and then, I'd have a cathartic break where those buried emotions surfaced for one reason or another. But usually, I'd return to my safe cocoon of denial and avoidance.

If you keep choosing the darkest version of yourself, you'll stay chained to the same pain you thought you were running from. Over time, mental illness can start to feel safe, as the disease state becomes intertwined with one's identity. It's the devil you know versus the one you don't. Potential effort to get better could lead to failure, and the thought of failure can feel like a crushing blow when you're already mentally ill. Change, especially the kind that forces you to confront uncomfortable emotions, is terrifying, and most people choose not to take that path. I remember a client once said to me, "So I operate at a 2 out of 10 instead of a 10 out of 10. At least I get through my day." He had essentially accepted his depression and was too afraid to let that darkness go. It had become "comfortable" for him.

For me, truly understanding my diagnosis of bipolar I disorder was critical, especially in conjunction with sobriety. That's what ultimately saved my life. I was finally able to see another version of myself: someone warm, loving, and understanding, a version that had always been within reach. I left Aileen on September 9, 2023, and in doing so, left that broken version of myself behind. That decision allowed me to finally break free from the cycle of insanity and abuse.

Following my psychologist's advice, I've kept little to no contact with her. As a result, my life has become peaceful and stable. She still tries to reach out from time to time, but there will be no response. As I've said before, federal prison looks safer and warmer than spending another moment with Aileen.

I eventually found sobriety from Adderall and cocaine, but when I arrived at Elle's home, I was still hooked on Klonopin and nitrous oxide. My excuse was simple: I needed something to numb me from the nightmare of living with Aileen, and those two drugs did the job. The only problem? I was taking upwards of 13 mg of Klonopin a day. If you know anything about benzos, you know that's an insane amount. I kept abusing both until one day, after a family court appearance with Aileen (an event that always shattered my mental stability) I completely unraveled.

That night, Elle and I had an argument. My brain, already softened by the drugs and rattled by seeing Aileen, couldn't regulate. I got loud. Loud enough that our housemate checked in to make sure everything was okay. I took it as a challenge and ended up wrestling him to the floor. Between the drugs and the emotional wreckage of that day, I escalated a situation that didn't need to go there. Just a sliver of contact with Aileen plus the substance abuse, and I hurt someone who didn't deserve it.

That night opened my eyes. The next day, the DEA showed up at my office, and I was arrested. But that night had been my breaking point, the moment I finally gave up on all substances all together. The truth is, I don't do well with any drug. If I can abuse it, I will. That's why I now stick strictly to my prescribed medication regimen, which helps keep me stable. It took 25 years to get it right, and that regimen is as follows:

- Abilify 2mg
- Atenolol 75mg

- Bupropion 150mg
- Clonidine 0.2mg
- Gabapentin 600mg
- Lithium 450mg
- Seroquel 400mg
- Sertraline 100mg

6 Psychotropic medications and 2 for blood pressure

Sobriety

Physical Exercise

Regular visits with kids and family, friends

Relationship with my sober fiancee

Regular psychotherapy

The Self-identified.

Regular sleep

Well nourished body

+

Acceptance, Honesty, Love, Self, True Happiness, Health, Stability

It took me 43 years and some of the most incredible experiences to get there.

Freedom on a Leash

Life after the arrest and arraignment looks nothing like the life I was living before. It's slower now – steady, structured, and, for the first time in years, somewhat stable. My days have a routine: fixed wake-up and bedtime, regular meals, and a strict medication schedule. I take the aforementioned eight medications, twice a day, to help keep everything (including bipolar disorder) in check. I don't touch drugs anymore, aside from the rare social libation.

My father asked me recently, "If you feel good and stable, why are you still taking all those medications?" It's a fair question. I explained that it's *because* of the meds and therapy that I feel good. Without them, a relapse is almost guaranteed. He got it – and I hope you, the reader, do too. If you're struggling and start a medication, like an SSRI (Lexapro, for example), and it helps you feel normal again after a month, *don't* stop taking it. The illness didn't magically disappear. It's just finally being treated and under control.

After everything first happened, my life was in shambles. In my mind, I had been publicly humiliated in front of the medical community. I shut down completely, cut off all contact with the outside world, and even changed my cell number. Eventually, I reactivated it on a new phone, only to be met with a flood of texts. Some people were angry, some confused, and others said things like, "I love you, man. You'll get through this." It was nice to see the support, but I didn't want to see or hear from anyone outside the apartment.

To make things worse, I was now on local news broadcasts, and around here, information travels fast. Word was spreading across Upstate New York like chain lightning. I was told that reporters said something like, "A 41-year-old psychiatric nurse practitioner of Albany was arrested on drug charges today and faces 25 years to life in prison, along with a $1,000,000.00 fine." Then they showed dramatic footage of a dozen cops raiding some random office building, squad cars lined up with lights flashing. In reality, it was nothing like that. A dozen DEA agents showed up in two unmarked vehicles – no sirens, no lights.

I never watched any of it myself. I couldn't. All I could do was pace around the apartment, peeking through the blinds every few minutes like someone was coming for me. My brain was in survival mode, and I became paranoid that the local cops were going to arrest me again out of nowhere and throw me in jail. When you're on probation, even something as small as getting pulled over for speeding has to be reported. I remember driving for the first time about four weeks after the arrest. A cop pulled up next to us at a red light. Elle was in the car with me, and I turned to her and said we had to switch drivers immediately because they were going to get me. As soon as the light turned green and the cop glanced my way, I pulled into a nearby parking lot. We switched seats. I just remember wanting to get home, crawl into bed, and shut it all out. I was twitching and shaking like I had Parkinson's.

Everything became exhausting. I wasn't eating, barely drinking, and my sleep was practically nonexistent. I was in a 24/7 state of anxious hypervigilance. At one point, we went to the AT&T store at the mall to get me a new phone, since the DEA had taken mine. I remember thinking, *What if the store employees recognize my name?* I had just been on the news. Even worse, what if a customer overheard me say my name and it jogged their memory? I was paralyzed with fear, but with Elle by my side, I felt just enough confidence to follow through.

By the grace of God, the girl at the counter didn't recognize me. I stood there, trying to keep it together, feeling like I was about to pass out. At that point, it had been nine days with almost no food and only minimal hydration. I'll say this – if you ever want to lose weight fast, just put yourself in a full-blown state of shock. You won't be hungry, you won't be thirsty, and you'll drop 30 to 40 pounds in a week or two, easily. Not that I recommend it, but that's how it went for me.

At that point, my life consisted of not eating or drinking and getting maybe three to four hours of sleep a night, pacing the apartment in a state of delusional shock. That pretty much sums up the first month or so after everything happened. But I still remember this one night vividly. It was Friday, and Elle made me a chicken pot pie from Trader Joe's. I ate most of it. It tasted incredible. My taste buds were so sensitive from the lack of food that it was like tasting something for the first time.

Then came another breakthrough: I went to the gym for the first time in about two months. Before the arrest, I had been going three to four times a week without fail. Let me reiterate how important physical exercise is, especially for those struggling with mental illness. You can't beat it. Exercise is superior to any drug out there (well, maybe with the exception of benzodiazepines). I remember calling my parents to tell them I'd finally made it back to the gym. They were so happy. It was a small victory, but still, forward movement.

I still had patients on my calendar for the next few weeks, though most canceled and about half asked for their money back. I remember calling some of the patients who hadn't canceled, and even went back to my office at the co-op workspace – the same place the DEA had dragged me out of – to see a few in person. Every one of them said the same thing: that this was a bullshit case, and if I needed help in court, they'd be happy to support me. It was reassuring to hear that, even though I didn't realize at the time that it would be the last time I'd speak to any of them. I still miss my patients; some of them had been with me for over a decade. I don't know what happened to all of them. I assume they found other providers locally, which probably accelerated how fast the news of my arrest spread. One of the big local mental health organizations was sending me four or five records requests per day, but I didn't have much to give – I had only just started keeping charts. While I was sick and addicted, I didn't document anything, which very well could have saved both myself and my career.

I still had January's income in the bank, which covered the car payment and rent for a couple of months. Elle started looking for jobs, quickly landing a remote position with a software company making $60,000.00 a year. I started Doordashing. It didn't pay much, but it got me out of the house, let me blast '90s' grunge on satellite radio, and, most importantly, sometimes Elle could come with me. If I started early enough in the day, I could sometimes make around $100.00 for six or seven hours of work. It wasn't much, but it covered things like gas, my cell phone bill, and groceries. My dad would often fill up my gas tank when I visited Connecticut to spend time with Lorenzo. Sometimes he'd even slip me $50.00 or $100.00 in cash for spending money. I had never really been in a position where money was a serious problem, so I appreciated all the help he gave me more than I could say.

Visiting Lorenzo was always a great time, but could feel draining at times. Between his hyperactivity and my parents' rules, parenting was challenging to say the least. Lorenzo and I had a strong bond, though – I was seeing him no less than two to three days per week. That added up to a lot of mileage. In the beginning, I had my Mercedes, which had around 70,000 miles on it. But when it got too expensive to maintain, my parents gave me a 2009 Lexus with 267,000 miles on the clock. It was my mom's old car, still a nice one, but it needed a new radiator and alternator (each of which ended up costing about $1000.00). So now I'm driving that car for Doordash as well as the weekly back-and-forth trips to Connecticut. I just pray it holds together until I get out of prison.

I found myself in a pretty good place – structured, sober, consistent, and committed to exercise. Elle was a big part of that, always being there for me, even when I was at my worst. I can say the same for Abbie as well. Supporting someone with bipolar disorder isn't easy; constant energy shifts can be exhausting. I still had days where I obsessed over what prison was going to be like, letting my mind drift into the darkest corners. On those days, I tried to distract myself however I could. I was never a big music guy, but the '90s grunge and alternative station played stuff I loved from high school, and it felt familiar. I found that listening to music, even while falling asleep, helped calm me down and pulled me away from obsessive thinking. In truth, I still can't fully grasp what prison will be like, what it's about, how to survive it. So, I end up tormenting myself. My higher brain knows it's useless to spiral like that, but the other 95% (the primitive brain) freaks out anyway. I have to really focus hard on staying positive sometimes, but it does get easier with time.

Once I began to come out of the severe shock (and I mean actual, physiological shock), I started to live life again, little by little. But this time, I was living with a much simpler, more present mindset. While awaiting what sometimes feels like execution, I've learned the importance of living in the moment. You never know what's going to happen next and living any other way just doesn't make sense anymore. There are still times when my mind tries to enter a state of derealization, which can quickly spiral into a panic attack. In those moments, I have to work to re-center myself in my environment. It's not easy but compared to where I was over a year ago, I now feel like I can handle the worst – because no one can take *me* from *me* again. I don't depend on anyone or anything for survival. I have myself, and I'm at peace with who I am.

Lockwood

Before my arrest, I strongly identified with my profession. Money meant everything, and I wasn't emotionally stable or available to the people who cared about me. While I wasn't using illicit drugs anymore, I had developed a serious addiction to prescription medications. True sobriety means complete sobriety – no exceptions. If you're an addict, you can't safely use any drug with abuse potential. In fact, I'm even addicted to oxymetazoline, Afrin nasal spray. It sucks. I can't breathe without it and have to use it every six hours. But I've found that there are healthier ways to cope, like exercise. The natural endorphin high from physical activity is unlike anything else. I know I just said it, but I'll say it again, and other providers will agree with me: you won't find a drug better than consistent physical exercise.

By the time April 2024 rolled around, I was finally feeling up to larger tasks and invited Elle to scale one of the 46 peaks in the Adirondacks with me. She had never done a hike like that before, and it had been quite some time since I'd ventured into the wilderness myself. I did research on the best mountains to hike in the Adirondacks, eventually settling on Hurricane Mountain – a 3,688-foot summit with a view that kept being described as "breathtaking". I couldn't recall the heights of the peaks I'd previously climbed, but this one sounded reasonable enough.

Elle and I planned our hike for Thursday, April 25, 2024, and the weather forecast was perfect. What I love about hiking in late April is that it's still cool but not cold, and the flies and mosquitoes aren't out in full force yet. Thursday morning came, and we were genuinely excited. I hadn't done anything like this in a long time, probably not since my last hike with Abbie when we were still together.

Elle and I got into the car and began our two-hour drive north, aiming to arrive around 10:00 a.m. We wanted to get there early to avoid any potential crowds and have a full day to enjoy the experience. Naturally, we got lost trying to find the trailhead for Hurricane Mountain. The spotty cell service up in the mountains made GPS almost impossible to use, but we finally found the trail and parked behind two other SUVs that had arrived earlier.

With a backpack loaded with water bottles and a small knife, we walked up to the sign-in sheet. Most trailheads have these sheets so that if someone gets lost, hurt, or worse, there's a record. I noticed a man and a woman had signed in about an hour before we arrived. I jotted down our names and contact info, and we started the hike.

The trail was stunning, with patches of crystallized water and snow still scattered on the ground like sequins. Everything was melting, so the path was muddy, making the hike a little more difficult than the descriptions online. Elle and I kept a good pace for a little while, stopping to take pictures and soak in the beauty of the waterfalls and nature in general. But as we reached the neck of the summit, the trail became very steep. We were literally taking one step at a time, pausing in-between to catch our breath.

Rounding a bend, we saw a man standing next to a fallen tree. Something about him caught my eye; he looked unusually short. As we approached him, I realized he had no legs, only prosthetics. I couldn't believe my eyes. He had already made it to the summit. He was incredibly kind, and we chatted for a few minutes about the trail before continuing on.

The whole way up, I couldn't stop thinking about him. This man had climbed a massive mountain on prosthetic legs and wasn't even out of breath. As Elle and I neared the top, we became completely wiped out. I made the call to stop while we still had enough energy to make it back down. I didn't want to be stuck on the mountain waiting for a rescue. We took a picture together and checked Google Maps, which said we were still 30 minutes from the summit. I didn't care. I was exhausted, and we had to call it there. The view, even from where we were, was still breathtaking.

On our way back down the mountain, we passed the man we'd met earlier. He was calmly enjoying the scenery, fully immersed in nature. We hadn't made it to the summit like he had, but when he saw us, he smiled and said, "You guys did that in record time." We went along with it. We both knew he knew the truth (no one could have made it up to the summit and back down in the time since we last saw him, let alone anyone breathing as hard as we were), but we were too embarrassed to admit it. We thanked him, our heads hanging in quiet shame. If he could do it, what was our excuse? The rest of the way down, we made plans to build endurance and get in better shape.

Lockwood

Once we reached the trailhead, we hopped into the car and headed to our next stop: the village of Lake Placid, where the "Miracle on Ice" happened during the 1980 Winter Olympics. The village itself is charming, filled with shops, hotels, restaurants, a beautiful lake, and tourist excursions. The massive Olympic ski jump still towers over the skyline. It almost feels like it never left the 1980s, but in a good way.

Elle and I grabbed a table at a tavern by the lake. Between the great food, the drink or two we each had, and the spectacular view of the lake, it was the perfect way to end the day. The hike had really tired us out, so we decided after dinner that it was time to hit the road (after a quick pit stop at a nearby chocolate shop, obviously).

The route out of the Adirondacks is a two-lane highway, and we ended up stuck behind a dump truck doing half the speed limit. It was a beautiful day for a drive, but I'm not a patient person (especially when it comes to slow drivers). I tried to push down the feelings of annoyance and frustration that had started to creep in, determined to not let one asshole ruin our otherwise-peaceful day.

After what felt like hours stuck behind the truck, a golden opportunity finally presented itself in the form of a passing zone just up ahead. My car had power, and I quickly passed the vehicle in front of us, then the dump truck, finally able to drive at the speed I preferred. Moments later, another car followed my lead, passing the truck and settling on a pace that matched mine. We both merged onto the highway heading south, and for the next 150 miles, we were road trip comrades. We passed slower cars in sync, kept the same cruising speed, and even dodged two speed traps together. When I finally pulled off at our exit, I rolled down my window and waved goodbye. The other driver did the same, and neither Elle nor I could keep from smiling. As annoyed as I was when it first began, the drive home turned out to be both beautiful and memorable.

That hike marked the beginning of what would become a busy but good summer. Even though every waking moment of every waking hour was still haunted by thoughts of upcoming incarceration, I continued to live. I had to, both for myself, and for my boys. As I was consumed by the weight of adulthood consequence, their childhood was unfolding in real time, fragile, fleeting hours no one could ever give back. I tried my best to make the most of every minute I spent with them.

Elle and I spent time that summer visiting Maine, New Hampshire, and Connecticut. We walked along the beach, explored tide pools, and went to improv shows, like the one at The Players' Ring Theater in Portsmouth, New Hampshire. We had a good time, and for the most part, my random drug screens didn't get in the way. Would I do a summer like that again? Absolutely, however, it won't be anytime soon since my sentencing date is now set for November 15, 2025.

Summer turned to fall, then to winter, then to spring. I busied myself with Doordashing, spending time with loved ones, and working on this book. The summer of 2025 snuck up on me. Even though I am acutely aware that I will be in prison by the time this season comes to an end, I wait patiently for whatever's to come. The thought of prison no longer scares me. I've made peace with it, and I have a strong support network behind me. In a way, I've "*8 Mile*'d" the situation (you know, the scene where he lists all of his "flaws" so his opponent can't use them against him in their rap battle) – I'm guilty of what I'm guilty of, and no one can use that against me anymore. I know who I am. Even my probation officer has told me I'm a good person who made some bad decisions, none of which define me. My release will not end my calling; it will expand it. I will still heal, but with a voice sharpened by experience and struggle and power reborn.

A Child's Love A Blooming Hope

With two months left until my sentencing, I hit a personal milestone: I had finally earned enough trust in my sobriety and sense of responsibility for Abbie, Elle, and my mother to feel safe entrusting me with the care of three children – Giovanni, Lorenzo, and Elle's daughter, Siobhan. I was extremely nervous; I could count on one hand the number of times I'd ever taken care of a child alone, let alone three, and even then, it was only for short periods. But the ladies were more than certain I could handle it, and that gave me the confidence I needed. Their trust meant more than I can put into words and marked a huge turning point for me.

I came up with a fun plan for the day: we'd start at the park, head to the apartment pool for a swim, and finish with lunch at McDonald's. I checked the weather the morning of the outing and was thrilled to see we had nothing but sunny skies ahead. It was June, school had just let out, and I was more than ready to make some awesome memories. I grabbed some extra sunscreen and jumped in the car to pick up my sons, Lorenzo from the nearby home of family friends who were taking care of him while my parents were on vacation, and Giovanni from Abbie's house. I swung by the apartment to scoop up Siobhan, and the four of us took off towards the park.

Castle's Perch was, by far, the best playground in the area. It was massive, clean, and new enough to have crazy shit like little ziplines. Once we arrived, I got the younger kids unbuckled from their booster seats and sprayed everyone down with sunscreen before turning them loose on the playground. The place was absolutely swarming with kids, but I never took my eyes off the three in my care. To ease any anxiety, I shared my phone's location with Abbie and Elle (who I'm sure checked their phones every five minutes). But the girls weren't nervous, and it reminded me once again how far I'd come in the last couple of years. There was a time when no one would have trusted me to pick up a pizza, let alone take responsibility for three beautiful children. Back then, I wouldn't have even dreamed of taking one child for more than thirty minutes – not just because others didn't trust me, but because I didn't trust *myself*. Back when I was still in active addiction, I knew enough to keep my distance and protect them from that version of me.

Adderall and Other False Prophets

The kids were having the time of their lives. Despite the difference in age, they always got along effortlessly and it was rare for the three of them to get to spend time together. In between making sure everyone stayed hydrated and spraying sunscreen as necessary, I had a realization. Yes, everyone trusted me, and that felt great. But I actually felt *good*. Watching the kids play was heartwarming, and the tranquility of knowing you're exactly where you're supposed to be, doing exactly what you need to be doing, is a feeling you can't get at the strip club, your dealer's house, or even in your own corner office. I was clean, present, and finally able to step into the role of a parent – something I had long feared I would never be capable of.

I worried the transition from the park would be tough and the kids might put up a fight, but it was so hot that they couldn't wait to go swimming. We drove back to the apartment so everyone could get their swimsuits on and grab towels and goggles and other pool stuff. Elle decided to take a break from work and join us at the pool (partially to help carry all the stuff). We walked across the parking lot to the pool, grabbed a big table with an umbrella, and watched the kids jump in. The three of them played so well together that other kids started asking to join. Before long, a full game of pool tag had broken out. I sat poolside, watching closely (alongside the lifeguard, of course), feeling a quiet sense of pride.

The kids played in the pool for hours until hunger finally caught up with them. It was perfect timing, as that was the next stop in my plan: McDonald's. We got everyone dried off and dressed again before piling in the car. At the restaurant, I was incredibly thankful that Elle was with us. The kids each had a different order, with multiple requests for changes or substitutions. She only had to hear everything once, and my jaw dropped as she successfully punched the insanely overcomplicated order into the self-service kiosk, including drinks, sauces, and special requests. She always had a mind like a steel trap.

After that, it was time for the boys to get picked up. Abbie's husband came to pick up Giovanni. In my sober, rational state, I appreciate just how good of a person he is and I will always respect Abbie for marrying someone who ended up being such an incredible stepfather to our son. We shared a moment together in the parking lot as I helped him with the arduous task of transferring a car seat between vehicles. He asked me if the kids tired me out that day. For a second, I considered denying it but he was just commiserating with me. So, I told him the truth: I *was* tired. We laughed, and he said "Yeah, that's to be expected," in solidarity before thanking me for spending time with Giovanni. It was a nice moment.

Our whirlwind day of fun came to an end, and it couldn't have gone better. Between the hot sun, all the running around, and the kids' high energy levels, I was wiped out in the best way. But I was also beaming with pride. I pulled it off, and everyone had fun (me included). It was one of those summer days you remember for the rest of your life, without a doubt. But to me, it represented even more than that. I had gone from a mentally ill, abused drug addict with completely fucked-up priorities to a full-fledged parent – someone who could plan and pull off an entire day of fun for three kids who, just two years earlier, probably wouldn't have even recognized me if I passed them on the street. It was a massive personal victory, one that made me feel more secure in myself (something I've always struggled with, as I'm sure you've figured out by now). The hug Elle gave me as she told me how proud she was was the cherry on top.

One place I received little recognition for the day was from my parents, particularly my mother. She had actually been pretty dismissive of any time that I was excited to share a parenting-related 'win' with her. When I texted her a few days earlier that I had gotten Giovanni a custom-engraved trophy for baseball, she brushed right past it, simply saying she wished she could've been at his game in person. That was it. Abbie, on the other hand, made an effort to acknowledge it, pointing out how special it was that I'd done something like that for Giovanni, and how excited he was to receive it. I don't know, maybe trophies at the end of the season aren't a thing anymore. But I do know it made me feel really, really good, and it stung when my mom didn't acknowledge it.

My parents should've known better. Just three or four weeks earlier, during a family therapy session, my mother had suggested I take Lorenzo by myself for nine days. I immediately buckled under the weight of it. The thought that I wasn't an adequate parent (or Lorenzo telling me to screw off because he wanted grandpa instead, which has happened before) was crushing. It hurt. I knew he was messed up from the trauma of Aileen, and I carried deep guilt for letting that go on as long as it did. Overwhelmed by that guilt and my own sense of inadequacy, I broke down sobbing in that session. I hadn't been that exposed in a very, very long time, and that kind of pain cuts deep. But maybe it needed to surface. I know I carry a similar kind of guilt about Giovanni, too (even though he wasn't tortured like Lorenzo was, I knew I hadn't been a good dad. To this day, I'm still grateful that Abbie made sure to keep him safe and away from me, even if I didn't appreciate it at the time. She's always been a great mom).

Throughout the day, I sent texts and pictures of the kids playing and having fun to a group chat with Abbie and my parents. I didn't get a single response from either of my parents. Abbie even made a point to tell them that I had all three kids on my own for the day – still, nothing. Instead, my mom sent individual texts to myself and Abbie about unrelated things (so, obviously I knew her phone was working).

Honestly, I could write an entire book on my mother, and each chapter would be more shocking than the last. And still, despite all of it, I love her. But sometimes I truly wonder what my mother really thinks of me. Lately she seems proud of me, and it feels like our relationship is better than it's ever been. But every now and then, she'll make an off-colored comment, and I'm left questioning everything all over again.

It's important to remember that my mom raised her three younger sisters after their mother left. She was forced to grow up too fast by being thrust into a maternal role while she was still just a child herself. That's how her personality was formed. That's why she is the way she is. Not evil. Not dark. Just deeply wounded, like the rest of us – only in her case, maybe a little more severely. My father is right: her heart *is* in the right place. But she doesn't know how to stop being the planner, the coordinator, the caretaker, the cook, the cleaner, and hundreds more. She's been doing these roles since she was a teenager, and by this point, the roles are so intertwined with her personality and sense of identity that they can't be separated. She's been the "identified mother" her entire life.

I think my mom does have some awareness of who she is and how she can be. When Abbie and I got married, she and her bridesmaids used my parents' house to get ready for the big day. I was with my groomsmen next door at my best friend's place. Now, my mom has a tendency to "run the show," and there was real potential for her to unintentionally make Abbie's morning more stressful than it already was. So, I pulled her aside and said, "Mom, you can't do what you usually do. You need to let Abbie and her girlfriends get ready in peace." To my surprise, she actually listened. She left the house that entire morning, giving the girls space to enjoy their time without any interference. I remember thinking, *Holy shit!* My mom always ran the show, and everyone usually let her. That was the one time she stepped back, and I was grateful. Abbie was, too. We both knew how hard that was for her, and we appreciated it more than she probably realized. When you're so used to taking charge and overseeing everything in your family's life, being asked to relinquish that control can feel foreign and scary. And on a day as important as your child's wedding, no less? Thank you, Mom, for trusting us to handle our own stuff that day and realizing how much it meant to us. We pulled it off.

I think we all have those fleeting moments of clarity sometimes. But it's uncomfortable, and the insight those moments provide is a gift that almost always goes unrecognized. We ignore it, pretend it never happened, anything to avoid the overexposed, vulnerable feeling of being seen too deeply (whether it's by others, or even just by ourselves). As I've written elsewhere in this book, discovering the self is a monumental and lifelong undertaking. It demands presence and experience. True growth often comes when we walk toward what we fear or don't understand; it's there that knowledge expands and identity evolves. The version of yourself that lives in your head is rarely the full picture, and it's scary to learn something about yourself that you can't reconcile with your existing identity. But it needs to happen if you're ever going to truly understand the self.

My mother remains caught in the same looping script of what she believes motherhood is supposed to look like, and any deviation from that would feel like crushing failure to her. These rigid loops prevent her from integrating new insight, which is why I believe her sense of self never fully developed beyond the trauma of being forced into a maternal role for her three younger sisters as a teenager. That role has simply shifted over time, from her sisters to my brother and me, to her grandchildren. She hasn't had to leave the role, just adjust it to fit whoever's in front of her. The day my mother steps back to care for herself would be a remarkable one.

Adderall and Other False Prophets

It's something we all quietly wish for, but we know the chances are slim. She was supposed to die in 2005 from a perforated bowel, but a world-class surgical team saved her. That should have been a turning point, a second chance, a gift of 20+ more years of life. But I can't help but feel she's squandered it by continuing to neglect herself in many of the same ways her own mother did for many years.

So yes, it's clear my mother has lived her life in the role of fixer – patching everyone else up while allowing herself to fall apart. It's a story I know all too well. Even when I was at my lowest, I still clung to the identity of a healer, of a psychotherapist. I let myself be abused while trying to fix Aileen and her kids. I'd been trained by the best caretaker in the business, my mother, and I was simply repeating what I knew (or what I believed at the time to be true). While my mother's addictions leaned toward cigarettes (in her 20's), Excedrin, Afrin, and alcohol, mine was Adderall and cocaine. The substances were different, but the underlying architecture was the same. I also mirrored my father in certain ways: I needed to always be hardworking, successful, constantly grinding. I worked far more than I needed to, spending any excess income not on stability, but on pointless material things and designer labels – all things that would eventually be destroyed by Aileen, anyway. It's embarrassing in hindsight, especially knowing I was neglecting to pay Elle at the time.

My day with Giovanni, Lorenzo and Siobhan not only proved to me that I could care for the kids but I was good at it and involved. Something else that I experienced was a feeling of love and support knowing I have connected with all 3 children on a deeper level. Because of that my unease regarding prison reduced a lot and more acceptance entered my life. I can and will do this because I have an army of people who love and support me. That's such a significant awareness that I never knew existed. And all those loved ones are there because I chose a life of sobriety and presence. Make no mistake, I relapse and become that awful version of myself, everything I mentioned will be gone. Every day I am reminded of how lucky I am to have what I have and am forever grateful.

Like one of my most favorite patients of my career once said, "I am 36 years sober however I am one sip away from day 1." Never forget you are an addict and with just 1 or 2 bad decisions you're gone, maybe even dead. Stay present, humble, grateful, live healthily, love and be loved and accept who you are no matter what anyone else says. Your story is valid and deserves to be heard, honored, and respected.

Conclusion

I didn't arrive here because of any one person, but I also didn't arrive here alone. The support I received along the way was invaluable. Sobriety and rediscovering myself were the true catalysts. For six long, dark years I had no solid identity. People like Elle and Michael reminded me that the man I once was still lived inside me. People like Aileen tried to bury him. She thrived on isolation and control, dragging me through humiliation, severing my ties with family, convincing me I was nothing. I became her Golem, bound to her ring.

But even in the depths of that ruin, I found the courage to rise. On August 23, 2022, my older son's birthday, I put Adderall and cocaine down for good. That day, it felt like angels sounded their horns. From there, the climb was brutal, but I refused to let Aileen break the new chance I had, especially with my sons waiting on the other side of my recovery. I fought, I clawed, and finally I said, *enough.* I left her. And in the rubble of who I had been, I found the one who mattered most: myself, Asher Lockwood.

Elle gave me peace, sobriety, and love. Even with prison looming, I have never felt freer. I see my sons every week. I'm engaged to the woman who stood by me. I've even traveled with my father, something I once thought impossible. Life is far from perfect, but it is real, and it is mine.

The work of healing never ends, but I am no longer afraid of the fight. You haven't seen the last of me I will return to private counseling, stronger than ever. My life experience is my power, and no one can take it from me.

I can't end this with magic words, but I can end with truth: stay loyal to yourself and to those you love. Don't let temptation or false promises strip you of what matters most. If you do what you love, you are already wealthy. Marry for character, not illusion. The right match will come.

Life is built on six pillars: health, relationships, finances, career, personal growth, and joy. I once had them all—and then I lost nearly everything. Maybe I had to. Maybe I had to be broken in order to be rebuilt. Today, my family tells me I am present, patient, and real. I know I am a father who loves his sons from the depths of my heart.

Lockwood

The world of drugs is a barren wasteland, a false paradise that only ends in ruin. I walked it, I lost myself in it, and I survived it. Many never make it out. I did. Sobriety is my freedom. Love is my compass. My sons are forever my legacy.

Maybe this was the road I was meant to walk—not to destroy me, but to prove that even in ashes, life can rise again. And so, can I.

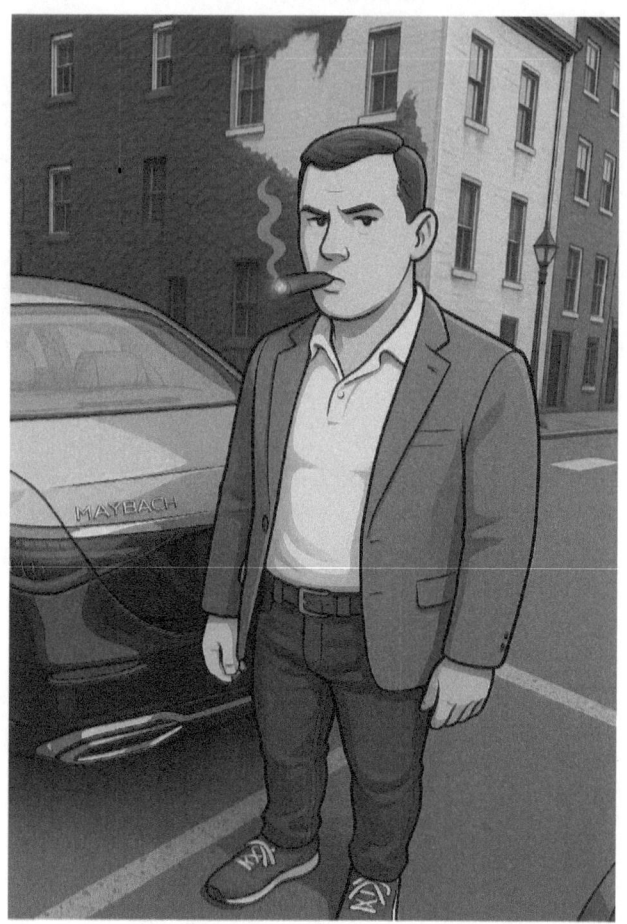

www.ingramcontent.com/pod-product-compliance
Lightning Source LLC
Chambersburg PA
CBHW021715120626
46545CB00004B/1578